C O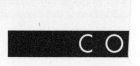

INTRODUCTION

My purpose in writing this book is to give you a sense that life can change for the better. When you feel expansion from the inside, everything in the outside world can work better for you. When you project optimism to the people around you, your positive feelings will be reflected back to you.

I've worked with people who could hardly move, and I've worked with athletes. I've learned that one's physical capabilities have little to do with one's sense of security, optimism, or despair. When we look deep inside ourselves and see the great power we all have, despair disappears and the external environment starts to change for the better.

In this book, I will tell you the stories of about thirty people who have worked with me to improve their health. Some of them were working to perfect the function of their already healthy bodies. Some had very poor vision, and every gain opened up more of the world to them. Others were suffering from paralysis and learned to increase their range of movement. Some of these people were optimistic at the outset, others were not.

My previous book, *Self-Healing: My Life and Vision* (Arkana, 1989), was the original version of *Movement for Self-Healing*. In this revised version, I've added more stories of recovery and described some of the exercise programs I used so that you can explore them yourself. If you suffer from any of the problems I describe, you will be able to see how these people got better — and how you can improve your health, too. In this book, I also explain the essence of my work in greater depth. *Movement for Self-Healing* has already helped people feel better about life. One woman, who read the manuscript after deciding to commit suicide, concluded that her life was precious and worth living.

This book is written as a series of stories. I felt exposed as I wrote it, because I present here the truth of my engagement with every person whose story I told. You may see yourself in some of these characters, or they may remind you of people you know. I hope that their determination, their challenges, and their triumphs will enable you to see how you can improve your own life. May their stories pave your way to a deeper understanding of yourself, to self-acceptance with love, and to more vibrant health.

PART 1

GROWING UP BLIND

CHAPTER 1
SAVTA: MY EARLY YEARS

I t was Savta, my mother's mother, who first realized that I was blind. This was soon after I was born — in Levov, Russia, outside of Kiev. Savta (*Savta* is the Hebrew word for "grandmother") observed me closely for several days; when she was sure, she prayed to God for the strength and wisdom to accept this new tragedy: another handicapped descendant.

Both my parents are deaf. My mother, Ida, lost her hearing at the age of three, following an undiagnosed illness. My father, Avraham, was dropped by his family's maid when he was one year old, and he suffered brain damage that left him deaf. My parents met at a school dance in Levov, fell in love, and married. My father's mother was so afraid they might have handicapped children that she slept in their room to prevent them from consummating the union. But as consummating a union is impossible to prevent, my mother became pregnant with my sister, Bella.

Bella was completely healthy. Thus made confident, my parents had another child five years later. I was born cross-eyed, with glaucoma (excess pressure in the eyes), astigmatism (irregular curvature of the cornea), nystagmus (involuntary eye movement), and cataracts (opacity of the lens). In short, I was blind. My father was busy launching his photography studio, and my mother, being deaf, felt incapable of handling the special needs of a blind baby boy and an active five-year-old daughter. So my mother's parents moved to Levov to look after Bella and me.

My earliest memories are exclusively of my grandmother. My grandfather had been arrested by the Communist government in 1943, eleven years before I was born, for using capitalist business practices in running a department store. He was sentenced to eight years in Siberia, and the government confiscated his large home and moved seven families into it. After only six months in Siberia, Grandfather was released when all the Polish-born Russians in the camp were conscripted to serve in the Polish Resistance. But when the Polish general in charge learned that Grandfather was a Jew, he kicked him out. Although freed by this curious circumstance, six months of abuse and hard labor had broken Grandfather's spirit, and he returned to his family a bitter man.

Thus, it was left to Savta to take care of me. When I was six months old, she took me on a train ride to Odessa — nearly 500 kilometers away, on the Black Sea — to see a leading ophthalmologist. Savta tells me that I loved the train ride and hated the doctor. The doctor examined me, with a group of resident ophthalmologists looking on, and declared that I would need surgery as soon as the lenses of my eyes were hard enough. Holding me in her hands, she smiled at Savta and said, "He is such a nice baby. Such a big head — a genius like Aristotle!" Then, turning to the doctors, she said, "We'll operate." One of the residents muttered, "I hope I won't be working that shift." After the meeting, Savta sought him out and demanded to know what he had meant. "At this age, his skull is so soft," he told her, "and this surgery would surely damage him." "We're planning to go to Israel in a few years," she told him. "Could we wait that long?" "Yes," he affirmed. "In fact, I think it would be much safer to have it done by a Jewish doctor." Concerned that harm might come to her grandchild, Savta packed our bag and immediately took the slow train 1,000 miles back to Levov.

Over the next three years, I became aware of my blindness. It was an uncomfortable, shadowy world — always dark. Many sounds were sudden and unexpected. I seldom knew where I was. The world was all hard surfaces and sharp edges, and only Savta was soft and tender.

Savta soothed and comforted me. The world seemed a little brighter when she was near, and I clung to her, listened for her, and followed her everywhere. When she went shopping or to the library, even though she assured me that she was coming right back, I screamed the entire time she was away. My mother, of course, couldn't hear me; even when she saw that I was having a tantrum, she couldn't stop me. Only when Savta returned and I heard her sweet, loving voice and felt her warm hug could I calm down.

Leaving for the Promised Land

WHEN I WAS FOUR, my family began the process of emigrating to Israel. Although we lived comfortably in Levov, my father was always in danger; among other things, his shop sold photographs of church icons, which were illegal under communist rule. My grandfather was all too aware of the dangers from the authorities. As Jews, my family felt that it would be better to live in a country governed by our own people.

At that time, direct emigration from Russia to the West was forbidden, so we first had to cross the border into Poland. We managed this thanks to the paper Grandfather had received when he was liberated from Siberia, stating that he was born in Poland (and thanks also, I've been told, to a bribable border guard). We had to stay in Poland for six months before we were permitted to leave.

In Poland, I had my first eye operation for removal of cataracts, the opaque parts of my eyes' lenses. It was excruciating, and I couldn't understand what was happening. Each night, Savta lay beside me, massaging my neck and face. During the operation, I remember waking up for a moment and seeing a doctor's face — his surgical mask and his eyes. I don't know whether I dreamed it or if I really did see him, but it was the first intimation that I might actually see; that image and the hope it instilled never left me.

After the operation, both my eyes were completely covered with bandages. When the bandages were removed, I was able to distinguish light, shadows, and even some vague shapes. People generally assume that blindness means living in total darkness, but after experiencing absolute blindness with the bandages on my eyes, I realized that blindness is relative and that I did have a little sight.

I recovered from the operation at home. Then, after six months in Poland, my grandparents, parents, two uncles, Bella, and I took our Polish passports and left for Italy. There we boarded the passenger ship *Shalom* and sailed to Israel.

I remember the crisp sea air and its salty spray, the big diesel engines that I not only heard but also felt through the deck, and the swaying of the ship, which made it difficult for me to stand. And I remember the light — the brilliant silver sunlight that I could barely discern reflecting off the Mediterranean. I stood at the rail and stared at the light on the water for a long time. One time when I was there, my grandmother put a piece of cheddar cheese in my hand. I remember holding it very close to my face and actually seeing my fingers holding it — and seeing a marvelous color I had never seen before. Grandmother must have noticed my eyes trying to focus on the cheese. "That is yellow cheese, my darling Meir," she said. I stumbled around the deck shouting, "Yellow cheese! Yellow cheese!" over and over to whomever would listen.

We landed in Haifa and settled in Morasha, a suburb of Tel Aviv. My grandparents and my uncles moved into one small apartment, and my family moved into another apartment in the same building. Father and Grandfather set about reestablishing their photography business in Tel Aviv.

Coping with Blindness

OVER THE NEXT TWO YEARS, between the ages of five and seven, I had four more cataract operations. In successful cataract surgery, the clouded lens is removed to allow light to penetrate to the retina. In my case, not only were the lenses not completely removed, but the operations created scar tissue that further blocked the passage of light. My vision showed no improvement whatsoever.

These operations were terribly painful and emotionally traumatic. In the hospital, I could hear children crying, doors slamming, and strangers speaking roughly. I was thirsty, and I hated the hospital smells. I was nearly always frightened. Savta was my only solace; she would hold me, soothe me, and massage me. We were in a hospital near Jaffa, on the Mediterranean, and she constantly reminded me to feel the refreshing sea breezes and smell the salty air. The one night I had to spend without her, I cried the whole time.

After five operations, my lenses were almost totally destroyed. Without glasses, I could see only blurred light and shadow, and with very thick glasses I could make out some vague shapes. Dr. Stein, a world-famous ophthalmologist who performed the last operation, pronounced my condition irreversible.

At home, I was angry and rebellious. The way my glasses concentrated light on my eyes was painful, and I would throw them on the floor and stomp on them. Although the lenses were too thick to break, I succeeded in wrecking the frames. I had persistent pain in my eyes, and I felt helplessly caught in a dark prison of shadows and outlines.

At the same time, I was aware of a part of me that was peaceful and that accepted whatever happened. Even in my most hysterical moments, I knew that things were not as bad as they seemed.

I was always using my hands to "see" textures and shapes. I loved to feel my family's outlines — their faces, hands, arms, bellies, legs, and feet. Although my senses of smell, taste, and hearing were unusually acute, it was through touch that I really explored and came to know the world.

Since my world was not visual, communicating with my deaf parents was difficult. I did not learn sign language, and at the time I didn't understand the importance of directing my lips at their eyes when I spoke. My father would grab my head, sometimes against my will, and pull my face upward to read my lips. His voice sounded like a leaky faucet dripping into a coffee can: "Boop bop blip blue blue blob." But I developed an ear for understanding him, and I knew when he was telling me, "Stop knocking over the damned lamp!"

Of course, there were many disasters. When my father and I went out together, I often got lost. I'd stand there and wail, but he couldn't hear me. I needed a Good Samaritan to figure out the problem and bring us together.

From about the age of seven until my early teens, I tried as hard as I could to be like others; I never accepted being "handicapped." When I wanted to cross a street, I could see well enough to know when the vague shapes of people began to move. Only when it was dark could I barely make out a red or green dot on the traffic light. Occasionally I'd just plow ahead, and drivers had to slam on their brakes all around me. I was bumped several times, though not badly, and quite a fuss was made. But I never used a white cane or a guide dog.

I went to the movies, and although my eyes didn't tell me much, I could hear the sounds and follow the plot. And I was never afraid of asking sighted people to fill me in. I even rode a bicycle, though I often rode it into walls, trees, and people. Once I unintentionally rode down a long set of stairs and banged my tailbone badly. I played soccer. Though I couldn't keep up with all the action, I occasionally got to kick the ball, and I was a good fighter. I loved to run around, but I fell down and bumped my head almost every day. Even today, people say I have a hard head.

The kids in my neighborhood generally excluded me. When I tried to join them, they played tricks on me. One minute they were there, and the next minute they were gone. They saw nothing wrong with bullying me; it seemed perfectly natural to them. I had to shout and fight to join in any game, and I had to work very hard to compete once I was in.

Elementary School

FINALLY, I reached school age. We lived in the suburbs, and the county provided transportation for all the handicapped kids who had to attend schools in the city; we weren't included in local schools. In my van there was one other blind boy, and there were several kids with polio. Every morning and afternoon, this group of blind and physically handicapped children rode into and out of Tel Aviv.

I was fascinated by the city. It was big and busy and noisy. I got to brag to the kids in my neighborhood about attending school in the city. I told them about games we played in Tel Aviv; anytime I lost a game, I'd say, "In Tel Aviv, we play by different rules."

In first grade, I took a class in Braille. The blind kids had an hour of instruction in reading and writing Braille at the end of each day. I found it difficult to sit in one place and concentrate on the raised impressions on the paper. The different arrangements of dots didn't make any sense to me. My first Braille teacher was an impatient woman who yelled at me and punished me whenever I made a mistake, which made it even more difficult to learn.

In Braille class, when I wanted to look at my fingers passing along the text, my teacher yelled at me, "You can't see the page anyway, so don't look at it!" This instruction to refrain from looking at my fingers — just to look straight ahead in order to fully concentrate on what my fingers felt — was especially annoying. It meant acting as though I had no eyes at all. By discouraging us from using what little sight we had, the teacher diminished the likelihood of our ever becoming "normal," and inadvertently helped lower our self-esteem.

There was another dilemma for handicapped kids. On the one hand, as a blind boy I was not expected to accomplish much; it was understood that studying in Braille was slow and laborious. But because of this, in order to compensate, I was also expected to work twice as hard as sighted kids. This, of course, was frustrating. Yet the more I was around "normal" kids, the more I realized that I could do whatever they could — and I was determined to do so. By the fourth grade, I was reading quickly in Braille.

When I was ten, we moved to Tel Aviv, and I had to learn my way around a whole new neighborhood. I continued at the same school, since that was where Braille was taught, so I didn't get to meet the kids in my new neighborhood. I was quite lonely, and I took refuge in books; I read voraciously.

Life at a "Normal" High School

In Israel, there was intense competition to get into a good high school. My teachers never believed that a blind boy could get into a good school, but my grandmother was determined to help me. She encouraged me to excel, tutored me as best she could with her broken Hebrew, and made sure that I believed in myself. I prepared intensively for high school, realizing that this would be a turning point in my life. With the help of my grandmother, who lobbied on my behalf with the principals of the top schools, I was accepted at the highest-rated school in Tel Aviv.

Despite all my fears and doubts, I was exuberant about starting high school. The possibilities seemed limitless. This was the excitement of the unknown. I had been encouraged, even pushed, to succeed by my grandmother and a few others who believed in me. But in high school I immediately encountered the same narrow views about the handicapped as I'd come up against before. I was forbidden to go on field trips, and I was excluded from premilitary training, which was compulsory for all the other boys.

In Israel, military training is a basic part of every young person's life. To be excluded was quite a blow. I appealed to the assistant principal, telling him that I was perfectly capable of doing everything that was required. It took several hours — I even pounded on his desk — but he finally let me take the training and go on the field trips. They wouldn't let me shoot a gun, but I could run as fast as anyone. When the other boys had to jump ten feet down onto a mattress, I was not supposed to do it — but I sneaked into the group and jumped anyway. I was able to push myself into every part of the training except rifle practice; the instructor was firm about that. Here again, I faced that unnerving contradiction: Because the instructor thought I didn't belong in the class in the first place, I had to do more than everyone else to justify being there. Although others could sometimes forget their uniforms, I always had to be dressed correctly. I didn't like being required to be anything more or less than everyone else.

In high school, I had to adapt to completely new circumstances. I no longer had Braille instruction; this was a high school for normal children. Many of the required textbooks were not available in Braille, and although some of the teachers tried to help me by asking other kids to read to me, I usually had to write to the Braille library and request that the books be typed out in Braille for me. This, on top of many long, arduous hours of study, demanded that I use my intelligence more fully and in different ways. I had to grasp ideas and facts quickly; I couldn't simply read about them later like the other kids. Since I needed extra help with reading and subjects like math, I had to be very strong in other subjects so that I could exchange tutoring with other kids. I not only had to get by, I had to excel.

I did well in most of my classes, but I was failing my class in Talmud (Jewish law) because the teacher was more interested in soccer and the girls in the class than in giving a coherent lecture. I depended on the class lectures because the written material wasn't available to me. My uncle Moshe, a well-known Biblical scholar who interpreted the Old Testament from a Marxist viewpoint, offered to tutor me. He felt that anything worth doing was worth doing perfectly. I would sit and read a page to him using two very thick magnifying glasses, one on top of the other; if I made even one small mistake, he would bend over and say caustically, "Pretty weak in this subject, eh?" It was difficult for him to sit patiently while I read so slowly, and it made me work all the harder to win his approval.

I also discovered girls that year, but at my first school dance no girls would dance with me. Considering my great expectations for success in high school, this was a terrible disappointment.

In the summer following my first year in high school, at the suggestion of my regular ophthalmologist, I was examined by the head optometrist at the Hadassah Hospital in Jerusalem. She had a lot of sophisticated equipment to examine my eyes. After studying me carefully, she prescribed two types of magnifying lenses that, for the first time, would enable me to see letters. One lens was a monocle of telescopic strength, with which I could read words on the blackboard a letter or two at a time. The other was a cylindrical, microscopic lens that attached to the frame of my glasses and allowed me to read printed words — also a letter or two at a time. To read, I had to put the book right up to my nose.

It was scary. Of course I wanted to see, but I already knew how to function as a blind person; it was frightening to think about changing that. Now I was forced to confront the belief that Braille teachers and others had instilled in me: that I couldn't use my eyes, and therefore I shouldn't try. At sixteen, I had become so set in my ways that it was difficult to take the next step.

During the summer, I tried to adjust to the close-up lens by reading a short novel. My uncle Moshe showed me what the letters looked like, and I learned quickly. It took me forty-five hours to read fifty pages, but in spite of the great effort and the strain on my eyes and neck, I was exhilarated. When I had begun to study Braille, it had been just as slow, so I patiently waited for further improvement. Sometimes I wonder how I managed to read or write at all.

During my second year of high school, I did all the assigned reading, wrote all my papers, and even passed the written tests without using Braille. I had agonizing headaches daily, and I often got nosebleeds from the strain. It was so difficult for me to write that I perspired heavily during tests. One teacher returned a bloodied paper to me saying, "You really put blood, sweat, and tears into this."

My math teacher treated me like an invalid, and expected me to be quiet and self-effacing. He offered me more help than I needed. He even asked another student to take notes for me in class. I told him that, after nine years of being helped with reading and writing, I wanted to do the work myself, no matter how difficult.

Some of my classmates began to treat me as a peer, but many continued to harass me. Once, when I needed assistance with a long geography assignment, I asked another student for help. He replied, "You have the book; read it." At first I resented this response, but after a while I realized the value of this lesson: I needed to be independent.

One day, the Israel Defense Forces Registration Department called. My father, whose deafness had kept him out of military service, said I should just show them my certificate of blindness so that I wouldn't have to go in for testing. This made me angry because, as I mentioned, serving in the military is an important part of life in Israel, and I wanted nothing more than to be accepted. When I went to the induction center for my physical, the ophthalmologist was amazed when I couldn't read even the first letter on the eye chart — with my thick glasses on! I was declared ineligible to serve.

Despair and Hope

AROUND THAT TIME, my ophthalmologist tested my progress in using the magnifying lens. She complimented me for working hard, but after examining my strong right eye she said, "Some kind of cataract is reappearing. I don't want to operate yet, but let's watch it closely and see what happens." I asked her, "Do you think my eyes can improve at all? Can any surgery improve them?" She answered, "No, I'm afraid not." I went home depressed. Even if I were to take a chance on more surgery, according to the doctor there was no real possibility that it would improve my vision.

And yet, deep inside, I had a different feeling. I was now able to see letters with a magnifying lens, and I was sure that I would learn to read much faster. I knew that the doctor must be wrong. I didn't know what improvements were possible, but I was convinced that a solution would come.

CHAPTER 2

ISAAC: THE FREEDOM TO SEE

Savta was having a difficult time. She helped Grandfather in the small shop where they sold my father's photographs, and business wasn't good. The shop was on a narrow alley near the Carmel Market in Tel Aviv, a noisy street with a few dingy restaurants — and a bad location for such a business. The lack of business also discouraged my father so much that he lost interest in taking pictures.

Grandmother's escape was through books. Though her Hebrew was still rough, she was well educated, and she read Russian novels endlessly. Her other delight was her grandson. Her love for me was something I can't possibly describe. Going to see her on Friday nights, celebrating the Sabbath together, being fed by her — I looked forward to it all week. The bread she sliced and buttered tasted so good to me that I thought it must be the most delicious food anyone had ever eaten. She would hug me, hold my arm, and ask how things were with me, how I was getting along in school, what she could do for me. Though I couldn't make out her features, I knew there was a glow of tenderness around her. It was the most exquisite delight to be loved with every look, gesture, and thought.

Every week, Savta would send me to a little lending library to exchange her books. I loved doing this for her. Miriam, the elderly woman who owned the library, always had a stack of books waiting for me. She sensed the love between Savta and me. Miriam always sat me down in her chair and talked with me while she worked. I could hear the smile in her voice as she said, in her strong Russian accent, "I know you must be a good student. I'll bet you're really smart." She appreciated the fact that I wasn't held back by being blind, and she especially liked seeing a blind boy coming for books. I felt like a courier carrying love between Miriam and Savta, and it was a joy for me.

A Fateful Meeting

MIRIAM TOOK AN INTEREST in health, and especially in massage and movement. She had recently helped a boy named Isaac, who was sixteen years old like me, overcome severe nearsightedness by giving him a book of eye exercises. Miriam told my grandmother that Isaac could now read much more quickly, and that I might benefit from meeting him.

When Grandmother told me about this, I wasn't too excited. I knew no one could help me read any faster, especially with my magnifying lens. But one day Isaac phoned me, and we arranged to meet at the library.

Miriam introduced us. Isaac impressed me as being a confident, sharp young man. He immediately asked me to take off my thick, dark glasses, and he looked at my eyes. After positively stating that my eyes could be cured, he asked who my doctor was. When I told him, he said, "She can't help you. She's very nice, and she means well and has a lot of experience, but she doesn't know anything about curing eye problems."

I was shocked. My first impulse was to run away. I thoroughly respected modern medicine, and I had never before questioned a doctor's knowledge or authority. Now this kid — who was actually slightly younger than me — was saying that my eyes could be cured and that my doctor knew nothing about curing eye problems! But as he continued to talk, I became more and more convinced that he was right.

I felt instinctively that Isaac might be able to help me. He promptly described all of my eye disorders: "Your eye muscles are very weak, which accounts for your cross-eyedness, right? Your eyes look astigmatic, right? And you've been operated on more than once for cataracts, which has left you with scar tissue and floating membrane, right? Right!" "This is incredible," I replied. And he said, "I can show you some exercises that will improve your eyes."

A week later, we met in Tel Aviv and stopped by my grandfather's shop to get money for bus fare. Isaac observed him intently for a moment; after we got on the bus, he told me in detail about Grand-father's heart problems, diabetes, and tendency for jaundice. I was amazed that he could know these things in such a short time. I later discovered that some people have this faculty: to look at people for the first time and not only pinpoint their health problems, but also sense how to help. Later I discovered that I have a similar ability, but at the time it was all I could do to accept the notion that this was possible.

I asked Isaac if he was a healer of some sort. I had heard about heal-ers who seemed to have a magic touch or some incredible way of healing people. "No, I'm not!" he snapped, "I help people heal themselves."

When we got to Isaac's house, he drew a diagram of my eye muscles and pointed to the weak or nonfunctioning ones. I looked at the diagram in a very strong light, but I could barely see the contrast of the white paper against the dark wooden table. I started to reach for my magnifying lens, but Isaac stopped me. "Stop relying on your glasses so much. Throw them away! I guarantee you'll be able to read without glasses in one year." I was shocked, but I immediately trusted that he knew what he was saying.

The first exercise Isaac showed me was called "palming," a method for relaxing the eye muscles and nerves. I sat at a table with my elbows com-fortably supported by a firm pillow, and I gently covered my closed eyes with my palms to prevent light from coming through. He told me to imag-ine something in motion. He said he liked to sit in class and palm, visualizing someone digging a hole. I found it difficult to visualize something I'd never seen. He also instructed me to visualize total blackness, and I had a hard time with that, too.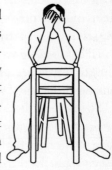

Isaac had learned these exercises from books Miriam had given him, all of which were accounts of the pioneering work of Dr. William Bates. Dr. Bates was an American ophthalmologist practicing at the turn of the last century who found through extensive and highly origi-nal research that the mind plays a major role in vision. According to Bates, physical or mental stress is the main cause of eye problems. When the eye relaxes, the correct cells of the eye are used, and vision is unimpaired. The key to Dr. Bates's teaching is the correct usage of the eye: using the eye the way it works when relaxed. Accordingly, he developed and taught a system of exercises for the eyes that are designed to promote their correct functioning.

Ophthalmology has since discredited Bates's findings and his exercises. I think the main reason for this is that practicing the exercises takes time, discipline, and patience; not everyone is willing to give that much to improve their vision. But I would have given anything in the world to be able to see. I was ready to do anything Isaac told me to do.

I felt exhilarated after my session with Isaac, and I ran to the bus and went straight home to tell my family about it. They were polite, but completely unable to understand or encourage me. I felt as though I were starting a new life, and I wanted everyone — my friends, family, teachers — to know. But only Isaac and Miriam could understand.

Isaac and I met again a week later, and this time he taught me "sunning," another important eye exercise. I would face the sun with closed eyes and turn my head slowly from side to side, making sure to complete a whole 180 degrees of movement with my neck and upper body. After I did this for a while, Isaac had me rest by palming, then resume sunning. I asked him, "How do sunning and palm-ing work?" "I don't want to tell you," he answered. "Just do it." I found this maddening. Still, from that time on I went up onto the roof of our apartment building several times a day to practice these exercises.

The following week, Isaac met me at our apartment. I was quite anxious, partly because he was coming to my home for the first time, but mostly because I was going to have my first date that evening. I had just bathed and dressed when he arrived, and he couldn't help noticing. "Hey, you look great," he said. This bolstered my confidence, and we went up to the roof so that I could show him my sunning. Isaac watched briefly, then snapped at me, "Okay, stop it! Just sit down!"

I was startled, and he curtly explained that the idea was not to flail the head back and forth, but to turn it gently and slowly. He reminded me to alternate sunning with frequent periods of palming. After we settled down a little, Isaac began to encourage me to relax and enjoy the exercises, and not to strain myself while doing them. Then he sat silently for half an hour while I followed his instructions, and for the first time in my life I knew what it was to relax. Though it was an unfamiliar feeling, it was wonderful. It even helped calm me for my date.

The session with Isaac turned out to be more satisfying than my first date. I must have bored her to tears with all my talk about sunning and palming. Calling her attention to my thick glasses and jittery eyes by talking about them so much probably turned her off. But it did help my self-esteem to finally have a date.

Once I began to do the exercises regularly and to really relax, I discovered how incredibly sensitive my eyes were to light. Even with closed eyelids, I could feel my eyes flinch from the sun; when I covered them with my palms, brilliantly colored stars filled the darkness, sometimes for hours. This disturbed me so much that I telephoned Isaac. "Don't bother me about that. You're making too much of it," was all he had to say.

"All right," I replied, "I'll look it up in a book."

"You won't find your answer in any book," he laughed. "It's really very simple — so simple it's a joke! But you'll have to find out for yourself." And he hung up the phone. I was frustrated to the point of tears, but there was nothing I could do. This was just Isaac's way.

I continued sunning and palming faithfully every day. I spent nearly all my free time up on the roof. Sunning became more than just an eye exercise for me; it was my life.

During our next session, Isaac taught me how to use blinking as an exercise. Dr. Bates discovered that opening and shutting the eyelids frequently in a relaxed way releases tension in the eyes, preventing squinting, keeping the eyes moist, and increasing blood flow to the eyes. This is the natural way for the eyes to function. When Isaac showed me the blinking exercise, I realized how much tension I had in my eyes.

Early in the summer, Isaac took me to the beach to practice sunning, palming, and blinking, and to show me several stretches for my body. I enjoyed this so much that, for the rest of the summer, I went to the beach as often as I could.

In mid-June, when the sun was highest in the sky, I especially enjoyed sunning and doing the other eye exercises. After sunning a lot, I would sit and palm for hours. At first, my chronic headaches and eye pains just seemed to get worse. But I learned that this was caused by the relaxation exercises, which allowed my body to finally feel all the years of accumulated tension. Realizing this, I continued the eye exercises and stretches even more religiously, and by August the pain began to subside. This was encouraging, and my enthusiasm for exercising increased even more.

There were times when my headaches were so severe that I couldn't move. One evening at my grandmother's house, I sat down in front of the television; as I strained my eyes to see, my headache became unbearable. My uncle Zvi, who lived with Savta, sat down next to me and started rubbing my temples. It was painful, but he assured me that massage could help dissolve a headache. And the headache did decrease. Though Zvi knew nothing about massage, he knew instinctively what needed to be done.

Once I learned that massaging the temples and scalp could relieve headaches, I began doing it myself. I discovered that, after massaging my temples and improving the circulation to my eyes, the outlines and shapes were a little less fuzzy, a little more distinct.

Expanding My Horizons

I HAD MY FIRST CRUSH that summer. I couldn't see my "heartthrob," but I imagined her to be very beautiful — even though I had no idea what that meant. My crush was a complete fantasy, but one thing was for sure: I was becoming very aware of girls: their sound, smell, shape, and touch. Whatever "good looking" was, everyone seemed to agree that certain girls were good looking — and that I wasn't.

When I was a child, the other kids called me "monkey," which in Hebrew has the connotation of extreme ugliness. I believed them, and today when I look at pictures from that time I can see that I did look something like a monkey. But Savta always thought I was fine looking, and I believed her more than the kids. I used to press my nose against the mirror and yell, "I am not a monkey! I'm gorgeous!" But when it came to a possible relationship with a girl, I felt like a monkey again.

Nevertheless, I was beginning to experience some self-confidence for the first time, and I was hopeful that I could overcome my handicap. But as my vision began to improve, I became reluctant to use my sense of touch. As a result, I began to bump into walls and people again, falling down stairs and stumbling off the curb into the street. Only Miriam seemed to understand the problems of this transition, and she encouraged me to use my sense of touch even more. She also taught me some basic massage techniques.

Miriam never told me much about herself and her training, but she did share a few stories. From the age of seven, she'd had many ailments, and she found that movement was helpful in overcoming them. She'd had two paralyzed toes and flat feet, and a famous orthopedist had prescribed a heavy boot and said that her condition would progressively degenerate. She was thoroughly convinced that his advice was not correct, and she cried for all the people he was "helping." Instead of following his prescription, she went home and did exercises in her bathtub, moving her toes in circles under the water. She walked every day and went on long hikes every week, and she managed to overcome the paralysis.

Miriam had also suffered from chronic rapid, irregular heartbeat. A movement education teacher had shown her how to move various parts of her body while he massaged her chest around the heart. That not only regulated her heartbeat, but taught her the subtle connections between different parts of the body.

After Miriam delivered her first child, she suffered a prolapse of the uterus. She told her doctor that, in two months, she would have her uterus back to normal. In fact, it took only a month of intensive pelvic exercises for her to move the uterus back into place.

Miriam made it clear that her deep understanding of the body was based more on intuition and experience than on technical knowledge. She respected the knowledge of doctors, but often questioned the way they used that knowledge. She had a strong intuitive sense of movement, and she loved to experiment with it, exploring all the different ways there are to move the body. And she loved to share her knowledge.

I had been rubbing my temples, but until Miriam showed me some techniques, I had never thought to massage my eyebrows, eyelids, eyelashes, and all of the bones, muscles, and skin surrounding my eyes. As I massaged away the pain of the headaches, they were replaced by a burning sensation in my eyes. My eyes were beginning to feel the accumulated fatigue from years of squinting and staring. Straining to see had kept me from blinking enough. Isaac explained to me the importance of blinking to rest, massage, and moisten the eyes.

I started eleventh grade with a confident, relaxed feeling about the future. The horizons I had imagined when I entered high school paled in comparison with what I now envisioned. Six months earlier, Isaac had said that within a year I would be seeing well — and I was determined to realize that.

After months of fanatically sunning, palming, and blinking, Isaac taught me "shifting," an exercise to improve visual acuity. In my case, it was also supposed to control my still-horrendous nystagmus. Nystagmus is an involuntary flutter of the eyes, which can severely impair seeing. Shifting helped me learn to focus on specific objects and introduced me to "conscious vision" — that is, seeing with the mind as much as with the eyes. With or without glasses, I could only see one big blur, so Isaac instructed me to look for details. For example, he said that when I looked at buildings, I should try to make out the position of the windows. He meant that when I looked, I should assume that the building had windows, and then try to locate them.

There was a tall building I passed on my way to the beach, not far from where I lived. I stood there every day for several weeks, trying to relax my eyes so that the nystagmus would slow down and images would appear. I imagined what windows might look like, and tried to find them somewhere I thought they might be. Finally, one Friday night, I saw them. I phoned Isaac to announce my triumph, but he was unimpressed. He told me, "Now look for the air conditioners. They're in the lower parts of the windows." Of course, I had never seen an air conditioner, and I couldn't guess what one might look like. But I practiced shifting for hours every day, and after only a week I was able to make out what I thought must be the air conditioners.

In this way, I slowly began to educate my eyes to see. Until then I had seen the world only as a single blurred unit. Now I was learning to divide that entity into details. By developing the habit of looking for specific things where they should be, I gradually activated my eyes and brain for the process of seeing. For sixteen years, I had been learning not to look, not to see, not to try to find anything. Everyone else would always find things for me. No one, including me, ever expected me to see. But now my eyes were full of windows and air conditioners, and my brain was beginning to function differently.

After six months of eye exercises, I no longer needed the cylindrical magnifying lens — only a pair of glasses. Furthermore, my astonished optometrist had to cut my prescription in half. Without glasses, I could see shapes, light and dark areas, and a little movement. With glasses, I was now seeing some shapes and patterns, the girls in my class, and even my own face in the mirror. I could make out the contrast between the color of my hair and my skin, and I could see my nose, lips, and ears — and even a pimple on my chin! Six months earlier, I couldn't see my face; now, when I looked really carefully, I could even see my eyes.

Resistance from My Family

IT WAS HARD FOR MY FAMILY to accept my improvement. I knew that my vision was getting better, but they still regarded me as blind, especially since my "doctor" was a teenager and my therapy some "meaningless movements." They tried to get me to stop doing eye exercises. This unorthodox approach seemed to threaten everything they believed in. How the exercises worked and what I was trying to accomplish were of no interest to them. Just as my Braille teachers expected me to accept my fate and learn to live with it, my family was afraid that my expectations were unrealistically high, and that I would just be disappointed later.

My grandfather was especially hard on me. He loved to be sick himself so that he could be the center of attention. He had every symptom in the book, though the causes were vague. He called them "attacks." Treating me as an invalid seemed to make him feel better. He would tell me not to carry heavy packages, play rough games, get into fights, or do almost anything that was the least bit dangerous. When I couldn't find something, he delighted in showing me where it was and how easy it had been to find it. "You're as blind as ever," he taunted me. "Your exercises are doing no good at all!"

Grandfather hated the fact that I was turning my back on "real" physicians. "This kid Isaac is even younger than you are," he scoffed. "Are you trying to tell me that a sixteen-year-old dropout can cure your blindness?"

I hoped that my great-uncle Moshe would be more understanding than Grandfather. He had worked hard to help me with reading, and he had always struggled for recognition for his own unconventional ideas. But he also couldn't understand how a boy of sixteen could be of any help to me, and he didn't give me much support, either.

Uncle Moshe had contracted throat cancer at the age of eighty, and I visited him regularly at the hospital. One day when I came into his room, he was asleep. I sat quietly and watched him with my limited vision. It looked as if a smile was forming on his face, and it seemed to me that his breathing was becoming more deep and regular. At that moment, I was able to see my uncle as if he were bathed in light. I could distinguish his closed eyes, the grey stubble of his beard, even the gentle rising and falling of his abdomen as he breathed. I must have sat there for half an hour as my vision grew brighter and brighter. I saw an old man near death who could dream about his life with satisfaction.

Then he began to wake up to the reality of his hospital room and his pain. The smile left his face, and I again had trouble seeing him. We talked quietly for a while, and I left.

The following day, Isaac was disturbed about something and needed to talk with me. This was rare, so I stayed and listened to him. Consequently, I missed my usual visit to my uncle. His wife phoned me and angrily demanded why I had missed going to the hospital. The next day when I went to see uncle Moshe he, too, was upset. He began to bait me: "Why is this Isaac helping you for nothing? He must be a homosexual on the make." I couldn't believe he'd said that. I was so disturbed that I ran all the way home and threw myself onto my bed, sobbing. It seemed that no one could see Isaac for his true worth. My mother came into my room and stroked my hair, soothing me. She was the first to see the improvement in my eyes, and although she had not trusted Isaac initially, she'd always thought he was a good kid. Mother's support at that moment was crucial. It was almost unbearable trying to convince the rest of my family that the work on my eyes was of value.

I continued visiting uncle Moshe in the hospital, and I knew that he was dying. We sat together for hours on end, talking about his ideas and mine. He never complained about his pain, and I found this inspiring. His spiritual strength and toughness kept him removed from the pain and from the sordid aspects of dying. He seemed to be living in another realm of consciousness.

The dreadful last days finally came. One morning, aunt Esther phoned to tell me that uncle Moshe was dead. I couldn't say a thing. But after the funeral, in spite of my grief, I felt a great peacefulness. While everyone else mourned, I felt like smiling. I knew that my uncle had not really died — only his body had given out. I felt that this was a wonderful secret that no one could share with me. His strong affirmation of life is still with me, and to this day I can still see him sleeping in the hospital with that peaceful, radiant smile.

A Low Point

SOON AFTER THAT, at my eye doctor's request, I went to Jerusalem to have my eyes tested again. While there, I visited my uncle Sadi, a prestigious engineer, and his younger brother, my uncle Zvi, who was also visiting. At dinner, my aunt Nayima, Sadi's wife, questioned me about

Isaac. I explained how Isaac supported himself, always buying and selling one thing or another, and told them many other things about him. Their questioning became more and more hostile, and only Uncle Zvi's girlfriend came to my defense. "What do you all want from Meir anyway? Why are you all so against what he's doing? I think it sounds great! If you won't encourage him, then why don't you at least leave him alone?" This led to an enormous family row. They told her to shut up and said that I was an idiot and a sucker. I was devastated. What a way to talk to a young man burning with zeal for a new way of life!

Uncle Sadi had the last word. "Look, kid, I changed your diapers and wiped your ass, so listen to me!" Then he drew what he thought was a picture of the eye and explained that, in my case, the pupils were missing and that I would never be able to see normally. He had no idea that the pupil is simply an empty space in the middle of the eye. My eyes were then so sensitive to light that the pupils were always contracted almost to a pinpoint. But my uncle just knew that there was something irreversibly wrong with my eyes and that I should forget about ever seeing normally.

This was an unhappy time for me. Isaac happened to be in Jerusalem at the same time I was there, and he took me to the hospital for my examination. He knew I was upset because my nystagmus, which had been improving, was worse again; nystagmus reacts immediately to stress. Because of this, I tested badly, and the optometrist decreased the lens prescription by only a little. When I told my uncle Sadi about the improvement, he said, "Is that all? Well, you're still legally blind."

"Maybe I should give up trying to convince anyone," I thought. "People don't want to accept the truth that my eyes are improving, even when it's right in front of them." But I knew it was important for me to convince others, especially my family, and I realized that the only way to convince anyone would be to show them.

Soon after returning from Jerusalem, I went to visit my grandparents. Grandfather was in bed with one of his "attacks." His hands and feet were icy cold. I had been practicing some of Miriam's massage techniques on myself, so I took his right hand and massaged it gently, moving all the joints to relieve their stiffness. I felt something like tiny granules under the skin of his palms and fingers, so I massaged them until they disappeared. Gradually, the color returned to his skin —

which I could see! — and he began to feel warmth in both hands and feet, even though I had only worked on one hand. "What are you, some kind of magician?" he laughed nervously. "But see how much better you feel?" Savta pointed out. "Okay, so it's better. But he is acting like a magician."

A Turning Point

AT OUR NEXT SESSION, a few weeks later, Isaac looked closely at my eyes and said, "I don't think you need the cylinder anymore." Soon after that, my eyes were tested by a doctor, and she confirmed that I no longer needed it, saying, "This is impossible. No astigmatism is correctable." But, in fact, I could read the chart better without the cylinder. So she lowered my prescription, and told me that after the next reduction I would no longer be legally blind.

Isaac said that I should also use these new glasses for reading. It was difficult to adjust to reading without the cylinder. In the beginning, it took me four hours to read one page. I needed very strong light, and even then I sometimes missed letters or even whole words. My mind wandered. It was difficult to concentrate for that long, and it was an enormous strain on the rest of my body. One time I tried so hard to read a single page that I suddenly threw up. "It takes so much time," I complained to Isaac. "So use your spare time," he shrugged.

He watched me read, and said, "You are missing words." Then he showed me an exercise to help me shift my eyes and move my focus from point to point, so that I wouldn't miss details. He explained that shifting the focus in this way enables one to make use of the macula, the part of the eye that sees the most clearly but can only take in one small detail at a time. By learning to focus on small details and developing the habit of seeing each detail clearly and separately, I was able to make use of the macula, and my vision steadily improved.

One day, I was playing soccer at school and got some dust in my eyes. It was extremely irritating, and I went to the school nurse to have my eyes washed out. But she just administered eyedrops and suggested that I continue using them at home. After several days of using the eyedrops, my eyes started burning so badly that I had to stay home from school. Sunning didn't help; in fact it aggravated the condition. I closed myself up in a completely dark room, and I lay down and palmed, with a towel over my face and hands, while I listened to rock and roll. The music kept me company, and the palming and darkness helped to relax my eyes and bring moisture to them. I was sure I was doing exactly the right thing. Then I began to blink, faster than I ever had before. At first my eyes grew moister because of the resting and palming I'd been doing, but then they became dry again. But something drove me to continue blinking for a long time, probably more than an hour. Eventually the itchy dryness went away, and my eyes began to tear profusely, washing away not only the dust particles but also the eyedrops.

I continued to blink, covering my eyes gently with my palms, and the tears continued to flow as if I were crying. It was utterly amazing. I palmed for two more hours, and then I tried sunning again. This time the sun did not disturb me, and my eyes no longer burned. From then on, my eyes have been considerably less sensitive to light and better able to protect themselves from dust and weather. The sunning probably helped a little, but I believe it was the fast blinking and the palming in a darkened room for several hours that produced those remarkable results. Isaac had been telling me that I didn't blink enough, and from that day on I began to blink a lot — so much so that people stared at me. My body had always been tense as a result of the tension in my eyes. The fact that I was able to recognize and respond to my body's needs clearly indicated how much my eyes were improving.

CHAPTER 3

MIRIAM: THE JOY OF MOVEMENT

One Sunday evening, Miriam invited me to her house for dessert. Over tea and chocolate cake, I told her about Isaac's prediction that I would be able to see perfectly in one year. She answered, "Even if you don't, even if you still have to wear glasses, it's far better to be using your eyes correctly than to go on using them wrong — to have eyes that are becoming more alive with movement and not just staring." She asked me about my eye exercises, and then she asked, "Do you work on the rest of your body also?" "Sometimes," I answered. "The calf muscles are connected to vision, you know," she said. Although my own calves were thin and my ankles and feet tense and contracted, I was taken aback when she connected this to vision.

As Miriam explained more, she became quite excited. For fifty-six years, she'd been exercising, always trying to help her body feel better. Every day, she discovered something new. Her enthusiasm was contagious, and I immediately recognized that I, too, wanted to try this movement therapy she was telling me about. I asked, "Why do we need movement, and what is the correct way to move?"

"We need movement because that is what life is about," she replied. "There is no such thing as a completely sick person — or a completely healthy person, either, for that matter. There are only those who move more and those who move less. Movement in the human body is continuous. Once movement stops, we stop living. There is either restriction to movement or freedom of movement, and a person can choose either. The correct motion is circular, rotating, and fluid, not angular or jerky. The round movements are beneficial because the basic cell structure is round, and our muscles want to move that way." She continued, her Russian accent thickening as she became more and more animated: "The human body has 600 muscles, but the average person uses only around fifty. Our potential is so enormous! We could use so many more muscles than we do!" I was in awe. I had never thought about this before.

Miriam began to show me some exercises. We stood up and moved our heels up and down, keeping our toes on the ground. Then we kept our heels on the ground and moved our toes up and down. We got down on all fours and moved our shoulders in a circular motion. We stood leaning with our hands against the wall and our elbows straight, shifting pressure from one wrist to the other to stretch our shoulders. Finally we simply rotated our heads. After that, my back felt much straighter and my head higher. After finishing dessert and talking for another hour, Miriam announced, "Meir, I expect you to be teaching me in two months' time."

When I went home, I was too excited to practice the exercises that night. But the next night — and every night from then on — I sat stretching my neck and rotating my head for twenty minutes before going to bed. I also discovered that if I did this stretch before reading, the words on the page appeared clearer. And when I did the shoulder exercises Miriam had demonstrated, my shoulders felt looser and stronger.

Every day after school, I closed the door to my room and exercised for an hour: first some stretching exercises that Isaac had taught me, then the exercises Miriam and I had done. I also ran in place, lifting my knees high and dropping my feet heavily to shake the tension from my foot muscles. Within a month, my thigh muscles had built up noticeably, and new muscles began to appear in my calves.

When Miriam saw me, the change in my posture was obvious. When I demonstrated the new running-in-place exercise I had discovered, she said, "I knew you would be teaching me." This time, Miriam taught me the importance of breathing. "You must always breathe through the nose, as in yoga. Your breathing should be deep and comfortable, always directed to your abdomen." She suggested that I go to the beach and do my eye exercises standing in shallow water; the movement of the waves would stimulate my foot and calf muscles. A new world was opening up for me. By the end of the session, I felt that I was receiving a precious gift of valuable knowledge about the body.

These "anticalisthenic" movements were not just exercises; they reflected an extraordinary attitude about the body. Rotating motions involve more muscles, and in a more balanced way than vertical or lateral motions. Miriam always tried to activate as many muscles as possible. She realized intuitively that many physical problems are due to a lack of movement, and can be relieved by learning proper movement. She particularly emphasized the importance of correct breathing. She believed that a lack of oxygen leads to disease.

With Miriam's guidance, I began to devote myself fully to the practice and study of movement, breathing, coordination, and the gentle rhythms of the body. Whenever I could, in summer or winter, I would go to the beach and stand in shallow water with the waves washing over my feet, lifting each foot in turn, and moving my head from side to side. It was pure bliss.

Yoga Finds Me at the Beach

ONCE, WHEN I WAS STANDING in the water with my eyes closed, an old man nearby shouted, "What are you doing?" I was taken aback and embarrassed, but I answered, "Eye exercises." "Oh, eye exercises," he said. "I can show you yoga exercises that are much better. C'mon."

I was about to reply that there was nothing better for my eyes than what I was doing, but he was already twenty yards away, so I followed him onto the beach to see what he would show me.

The old man's face was brown and wrinkled, and what little hair he had was white. But his body looked very strong — many years younger than his face. "My name is Shlomo," he said. Then he showed me a very gentle exercise that I liked immediately. With my left hand, I held the back of my head and moved it from side to side, while my right hand pressed firmly against my forehead. This exercise loosened my neck and massaged my forehead at the same time, which was very stimulating for my eyes. Shlomo excused himself after this one exercise, but he said that he came to the beach every day and told me to look for him.

That afternoon, I saw Miriam and asked her what she thought of yoga. "It's okay," she replied, "as long as you don't do it mechanically or passively. If you can do it actively and with awareness, it is wonderful."

The next day, I found Shlomo leading a group of older men and women in yoga exercises. When someone had a problem, he would correct it. His stretches seemed unusual to me at first, but I came to see that they were actually simple and reflected his clear understanding of the body. I was quite weak and stiff, and I found the exercises difficult to do, but I could see the sense of them and I joined in gradually.

Shlomo said to me, "You know, there's no trick to it — no secret. There's not even any strenuous effort. It's simply a matter of moving every part of the body, from the tips of the toes to the crown of your head." That was exactly what Miriam had said!

Shlomo showed me a number of exercises that he found suitable for his body. He said that, although his back was slightly stiff, he could barely bend it at all before he began exercising. He'd always had a tendency toward aches and pains because his spinal disks had deteriorated from hard physical labor as an Israeli pioneer. Yet he now appeared to have the strength and flexibility of a thirty-year-old; he could move each vertebra separately as he bent over.

Shlomo was pleased by my interest in his work, and he showed me many exercises. He moved his arms in circles: first the entire arm, then just the forearm. He clasped his hands with one arm behind his head and the other behind his back. While clasping his hands, he bent his upper body forward and rotated his spine. Then he lay stretched out on one side and, leaning his head on his hand in what he called "The Philosopher's Position," brought one knee to his forehead, then bent that leg backward and touched the back of his head with his foot. Lying on his back, he lifted one knee to his chest, then lifted his head with his hand to touch the knee to his forehead. This old man's flexibility was impressive!

Shlomo told me that he did many other exercises every day, and that one must do an exercise twenty or more times consecutively for it to really activate the joints and muscles.

Shlomo and I spent most of that summer together, stretching and doing yoga. One day, he took me to a class in Tel Aviv given by Moshe Feldenkrais, a pioneer in the field of therapeutic movement. I learned some valuable things there. Like Miriam, Feldenkrais recognized that any movement should take into account the whole body, and that the most effective movement is not strenuous, but gentle.

Shlomo made a great contribution to the foundation of my ideas about exercise and bodywork. I was only seventeen and he was seventy-seven, and I learned so much from him. His flexibility and innate sense of movement made a deep impression on me.

What a wonderful summer it was, climaxing the most important year of my life! First, Isaac taught me eye exercises and told me that I would see without glasses. Then Miriam taught me gentle movement and breathing. And now Shlomo was showing me stretches to loosen and strengthen my body even more. I knew I was at a crossroads.

CHAPTER 4

MY FIRST PATIENTS

One autumn day during my last year of high school, while I was practicing sunning exercises after lunch, a classmate named David came over and asked what I was doing. I told him about the exercises, and about how much they'd helped me. David was one of the few students who had shown a positive interest in my work, and he'd always been pleasant to me. A few times, he'd even asked for my advice about some health problems.

David told me that his girlfriend, Adina, the prettiest girl in our class, was having such severe headaches that she was hardly able to sleep. She was also having frequent nightmares and irrational fears. I recommended that they talk with Isaac, and offered to arrange a meeting. Not long afterward, David and Adina came to my house for a successful session with Isaac. At the end of the meeting, Adina thanked me for helping her. I said, "The only thanks I want is for you to work on yourself." I was really happy to help, even if only indirectly.

On My Own

BUT A FEW DAYS LATER, Isaac disappeared for what turned out to be months. On the best of occasions, he was only available when he felt like it, but now he was completely abandoning both Adina and me.

During this time, I felt that I really needed guidance and direction. But Isaac wasn't available. In spite of my concern and my hurt feelings, his influence and example remained strong; I continued to feel as if he were guiding my efforts.

Sometimes I would go down to Allenby Street, where all the felafel stands were, and have a felafel. It reminded me of Isaac, because he was crazy about felafel. Along one side of the street was a row of felafel shops, each run by a different family. They made their felafel according to closely guarded secret recipes, mixing garbanzo flour with spices, oil, and other ingredients, then shaping the mixture into patties and frying them. The felafel was then stuffed into pita bread with vegetables and sesame butter, and you could either take it out or eat it there at small tables. There were always long lines at the booths.

I had no special craving for felafel, but being on Allenby Street made me feel connected to Isaac somehow. It reminded me of the long hours we used to spend there, usually accompanied by some girl he'd brought along, talking about all kinds of things. Although it wouldn't actually occupy much of the conversation, it seemed to me that we were always talking either about my eyes or about health in general — subjects in which I was most interested, of course. I drank in everything Isaac said with tremendous thirst, and struggled to read his expression to understand the meaning behind his words. The things he said were of great importance to me, and had enormous influence on me. I remember him saying, "Every disease is curable. Your eye problems, Meir, can definitely be cured, in spite of all the operations and the thick glasses you've worn all your life. Your eyes will soon be cured and you will see perfectly."

Though I was unhappy about being abandoned by Isaac, I was particularly upset about his treatment of Adina; I felt that he should have continued to see her at least until she showed some improvement. One day I went to Miriam's library, and Adina happened to be there. She seemed pleased to see me, but her condition was apparently getting worse, and she'd been in a lot of pain. Miriam overheard us talking and offered to show Adina some exercises. But before she did so, she said, "Why doesn't Meir show you some exercises that he knows?" Adina was immediately interested, but I was hesitant. I finally allowed myself to be persuaded to see her at her home the following week. After she left, Miriam said, "I won't work with you anymore unless you work with Adina."

Every day that week, I went to the library to learn some exercises from Miriam that could help alleviate Adina's headaches. Then I went home and tried them out. Finally, I went to Adina's house and taught her several exercises that I thought would be especially good for her. She began doing them faithfully, and I returned once a week to work with her. After a month, her headaches diminished considerably.

During my sessions with Adina, I learned that she was taking anti-depressant drugs prescribed by a psychiatrist. I told her that I was afraid the drugs might hurt her and that I thought she should stop taking them. When she told her parents this, they were enraged.

Miriam felt that I shouldn't antagonize Adina's parents; Miriam had great respect for parents, and would never do anything against their wishes. The day after this incident, she suddenly announced that she would no longer be available to help either Adina or me for two reasons. "First, I'm working too hard already. The second reason I can't tell you. You'll have to figure it out for yourself."

First no Isaac, and now no Miriam. I was stunned! What could I tell Adina? She had been eagerly doing her exercises, and she'd placed a great deal of trust in Miriam and me. I saw Adina in school the next day and tried to make something up, but the truth poured out. Adina was shocked and nearly speechless. "But Miriam promised!"

Adina was on my mind all day. As I was doing my exercises at home in the afternoon, I concentrated on her head and shoulder tension. I began to feel as if my body became hers, experiencing her tension from within. I lay face down on the floor, lifted my upper body, and rotated my head and shoulders. This released a lot of tension and made that area feel looser and stronger. This was a new exercise for me, and I was sure it would be good for Adina. I devoted the rest of the afternoon to finding exercises for her.

The next day, I showed the exercises to Adina with an apology: "I'm not very good at this." "Don't say that," she protested. "I think you're as good as Isaac and Miriam. In fact, you're better; you're still here. You have a talent, Meir, and I trust you." Adina was my first patient, and this compliment was a big encouragement for me.

Over the next few months, Adina's headaches and insomnia disappeared completely. I felt a tremendous sense of achievement. Adina helped me believe in myself. She reaffirmed what I felt inside, and this was deeply satisfying.

One day, four months since I'd last seen him, I unexpectedly bumped into Isaac. In fact, I didn't see him as we passed on the sidewalk; he saw me. Isaac slapped me on the back and said, "Still not talking to me, eh?" as if I'd abandoned him. But I was too glad to hear his voice to be angry.

We talked as he waited for the bus, and he told me, "You know, Meir, I feel that my work with you has been important, not just because of what it will do for you, but because I know you will help other people. You have a very good instinct and your sense of touch is already better developed than some people with twenty years of experience. I expect you to become a great teacher."

I went home filled with inspiration. This brief encounter changed my life. I had dreamed of becoming a diplomat, or maybe a foreign minister. But when Isaac suggested that I work as a healer, I knew he was right. His confidence awakened in me an awareness that had been dormant: The work I was doing could become my life's work.

An Ally and a New Challenge

DURING THE SAME WEEK when Miriam severed my dependence on her, she also stopped working on my friend Dorit, a polio victim who'd had thirteen operations on her legs. Miriam had met Dorit when she was about to have her fourteenth operation, and convinced her to try exercising instead. Miriam then introduced Dorit to me so that we could encourage and learn from each other. Though our problems were different, we felt a strong bond; we were working together on "incurable" disabilities. We had to conquer our negative attitudes, and then conquer the problems themselves. We needed to decide not to be cripples.

Dorit had excruciating pain in both legs. The operations had caused a lot of damage. At Miriam's suggestion, Dorit worked on herself for two hours a day, and sometimes went on for another three or four hours after that. She did Miriam's exercises as well as some she found in books and some she invented herself. Dorit wanted to become a physical therapist, but her parents found this unsuitable for a proper Orthodox Jewish woman; they wanted her to marry and settle down. This was frustrating for her, and I listened to and supported her.

In spite of the pain, Dorit loved walking, and we often walked together. One day, we walked quite a distance to pick up a new pair of specially designed orthopedic shoes. Dorit limped a little on the way home, but her walking wasn't too bad. At home, she said, "It's not my muscles that kept me going; they're too tired. It was just will power. That was farther than I've ever walked before." Dorit didn't just want to walk without a cane. She didn't even just want to climb mountains. She wanted to walk exactly like other people, and she would do whatever was necessary to achieve this.

A young man named Eli, who was severely crippled with muscular dystrophy, was getting a lot of publicity in Israel at the time. He was trying to get accepted into the army to show that someone severely handicapped could make a contribution to his country. He argued that he could serve Israel with his intelligence, even though his body was paralyzed. I supported his cause, but it was Dorit who thought to phone him and offer help.

Dorit told him that he was fighting too much against society and not enough against his muscular dystrophy. Eli responded that there was nothing he could do about the disease, and that he was in good shape compared to many others who had his kind of muscular dystrophy. Dorit insisted, "There is a lot you can do about your disease if you want to." I also spoke to him and managed to interest him in the possibility that we might be able to help him.

A few days later, Dorit and I went to Eli's house in Tel Aviv. Eli had a handsome and sensitive face, but his body was more deformed than either Dorit or I had ever seen. His head flopped onto one of his shoulders, and many of his bones were out of place.

"Are you shocked by the way I look?" he asked. "No, I'm not," I answered, and I wasn't. I was too busy thinking about what we could do to help him.

"When I was born," Eli told us, "the doctors said I wouldn't live three years. My vertebrae are totally out of alignment; they curve both left and right. My ribs are completely twisted around, and that shoves my heart over by my right armpit. It's funny when these famous doctors examine me with their stethoscopes and can't even find my heart!" He said that his body temperature was high and his palms and the soles of his feet were usually sweaty. He suspected that this warmth had kept him alive.

I explained our work to Eli: "Rotating motions help all the muscles that are involved in the movement to work together, and to work and rest alternately. We can activate all your muscles." Then Dorit told him about the benefits of massage for strained, tight, weak, or injured muscles, saying, "The most important thing is to adjust the touch for your body." Eli told us that, although he'd had physical therapy and hydrotherapy, his back had never been massaged. Dorit insisted that his whole body needed massage, and Eli promptly assented. When Dorit and I left Eli's house, we were in complete agreement. Dorit felt that, of the two of us, she knew best how to work on his body, and she hinted at this several times. I didn't mind; in fact, I was happy to work with someone who felt so knowledgeable and confident.

A week later, Dorit and I began to work with Eli. Dorit initially asked Miriam for advice on how to work with him, but after a short time she took off on her own. "Now the world has the Dorit Method," Eli joked.

Eli's arms and legs were crooked, and he couldn't straighten them out by himself. His muscles were thin and his hands were so weak that his skinny fingers curled up on his palms. His ribs were completely misshapen, bulging out in some places and caving in at others. It was curious that I could see him so well; it was probably due to my great interest.

After only two sessions, Eli was able to hold his head more or less upright for about ten minutes, and he could move heavy books around on his desk. Even the muscles of his fingers and upper arms showed a little more substance.

Dorit and I began to work on Eli at different times, and we also trained the members of his adoptive family to work on him. Eli's improvement, though slight, was a great encouragement to me.

Then suddenly, out of the blue, Dorit told me, "Eli and I are going to get married." I couldn't believe my ears! It wasn't Eli's crippled condition that disturbed me, but the fact that Dorit was eighteen, and that they were deciding to marry after an acquaintance of only four weeks. I burst out laughing and said, "You're joking!" But they weren't. I was stunned and skeptical, but my reaction was mild compared to the others they encountered. Her parents were horrified at the idea, and refused to even listen to her. They were extremely religious people, and had not even imagined that Dorit would be allowed to choose her own husband — let alone make the choice she'd made! Even Miriam was appalled: "Doesn't she know he's going to die in a couple of years? What kind of marriage will that be?"

But the marriage never took place; Dorit's parents managed to stop it. The matter was finally decided by her rabbi, who found her a rabbinical student from New York City to marry. Despite her rebellion against her parents, Dorit could not go against the rabbi's wishes; he was the very spirit of her religion. For three sleepless nights, she agonized over the decision, and finally decided not to marry Eli.

Eli was despondent, but after a while he recovered and I began to work on him by myself. It was encouraging to see him get stronger. After only two months, he could hold his head up for an hour. I knew that he could be helped, and that within five years he would be able to walk if he worked on himself.

Unfortunately, Eli's emotional roller coaster continued. Just four months after recovering from Dorit's abandonment, he announced his plans to marry Tsippi, his adoptive sister. Their adoptive mother gave them two hours to pack and leave. They stayed at my house for a week until they found a place to live. Three days before the wedding, Tsippi's biological mother came to their apartment to try to kill Eli, shouting that her daughter would not marry such a cripple. The police put Tsippi's mother in custody, and she remained in jail until after the marriage.

It wasn't long before Eli lost interest in my treatments. When I came to work on him, it was apparent that he hadn't exercised between visits. Although his body had improved remarkably in a short time, he wasn't willing to go beyond that point. I had to accept this decision. I could only assist him; I couldn't magically heal him.

My Own Progress

MEANWHILE, I continued to make progress with my eyes. My goal was to be able to read without glasses, and I spent hours each day working toward this goal. I had stopped using the cylindrical microscopic lens some months before, and was reading with only my new glasses. It took nearly four hours to read a page that I could have read in ten minutes with the cylinder, but I was determined.

Sometimes my eyes grew tired from trying to read, so I would take my glasses off and put my nose right down on the page. To my astonishment, sometimes the letters would appear! Then I would try to guess what the word containing those letters might be and, to my amazement, there would be the whole word. But I remembered that Isaac had told me to read only with the glasses, so I put them back on. At times I took my grandmother's glasses, which had a much weaker prescription, and managed to read for a while even with them. But I found the challenge of reading without glasses irresistible, and I tried it more and more frequently.

My eyesight had begun to develop, and the external world was taking shape for me. At the same time, a decision gradually formed in my mind, becoming firmer and firmer: One day, I would be able to see clearly what was around me. Isaac had promised that I would have good eyesight in six months or so. That wasn't quite the way it turned out, but my eyes improved enough that I was not disappointed. One is not always aware of improvement while it is taking place, but I could tell that my eyes were getting stronger and would continue to do so. For one thing, I was reading much more easily with my special magnifying lens. Not only that, but I had begun to read with both eyes. My weaker, left eye no longer added a blurred image to my field of vision as I focused on each letter; it had become strong enough to take an active role in the vision process. I think that the nerve centers in my brain had probably also begun to adjust to the new, improved situation. My nystagmus condition, which had been quite bad, had lessened enough that I could control my eye movements somewhat. I was on my way to a completely different life.

I never stopped working on my eyes, even while sitting in classes. Listening to the teacher, I would shift my eyes from one loudspeaker to the other in the front corners of the classroom. I was constantly moving my eyes from point to point, for by now they were strong enough to benefit from this. I often palmed, especially during music class, where I could palm for forty-five minutes while listening to the lectures and symphonies.

One day my geography teacher asked me, "How do you expect to get a good grade if you're always doing eye exercises and not listening to me?" I told her that I was doing both at the same time, but this only flustered her. "How can you move your eyes and still hear my voice?" She must have realized how ridiculous the question was, especially when I pointed out that people use their eyes and ears at the same time all day long. Even if they were a little disturbing to my teachers and classmates, the exercises were a necessity to me. And a few teachers and students accepted what I was doing.

While still in high school, I decided to take a course from a vocational massage school in order to improve my bodywork techniques.

Unfortunately, all I learned was that Miriam knew more about massage than the instructors. They taught us a rigid program of techniques; some were useful, but most were not. They never mentioned paying attention to what an individual person really needs. They didn't teach, for example, what position the therapist's body should be in while working on a patient, and they never mentioned different types of touch for different bodies or the importance of the therapist's own relaxation and presence. Though I took the course for six months, I decided not to apply for the massage certificate that was offered. The main thing I gained from this course was a sense of confidence in what I was already doing. I also enjoyed the free massages I got when we all worked on each other.

By that time, I was using massage and movement to help several people — people I met on the beach, people Miriam sent, and friends of those people. Some of them felt strongly that they should pay me for my work. I had always refused, but after I completed the massage course I began to feel that it might be alright to accept payment.

Danny

A FEW WEEKS before my high-school graduation, Miriam called me. I was always happy to hear from her. She told me about a young man named Danny; he had recently arrived in Israel from Iran, and was having difficulty walking because of progressive muscular dystrophy. She said that his condition was severe, and she hoped I would see him.

A few weeks later, Danny called to ask if I could do anything for him. "My situation looks bad. All the doctors say there is nothing that can be done. Are you sure you can help me?" I told him about Eli who, at that time, was still improving steadily. Danny was quite impressed, so we set a time to meet.

The first time I saw Danny, I thought he was just a boy. I was only a year older and a little taller, but he seemed about half my size. His face wore an expression of distress, and his hands trembled, yet there was something charismatic about him. He was honest and direct, and full of intensity. During the next few years, Danny became not only my patient, but also my teacher and my closest friend.

I examined Danny and tested the strength of his legs. All of his toes curled upward because the muscles weren't strong enough to hold them in place. His legs were very thin, and the thighs were even thinner than

41

the calves. His stronger leg, which bore most of his weight when he stood and walked, was hard with contracted muscles. His fingers were as thin as a baby's, and his arms were almost fleshless; he could lift them only as high as his chest. His shoulders were so emaciated that if you pulled on his arms you could dislocate his shoulders. His face was thin, and there was something miserable and frightened in his expression.

Muscular dystrophy is a progressive disease that causes the muscle fibers to degenerate. Like Eli, Danny was diagnosed with the Duchenne type of muscular dystrophy, which leads to a slow death, with the patient eventually becoming too weak to breathe. Danny's symptoms, however, were not as severe as Eli's.

Danny and I discussed a treatment strategy, and I told him, "You can definitely be cured." At the time, I was relying more on my intuition than my knowledge. He looked at me in amazement. He wasn't sure he could believe me, but even the possibility of a reprieve from degeneration and death seemed like salvation to him.

During our first two sessions, I did all the work. I showed Danny how to rub his hands together to warm them, but at first he was only able to do this a few times before becoming exhausted. I massaged his fingers to stimulate them and increase the circulation. I worked for many hours on his arms and shoulders, gently massaging and rotating them. After several sessions, Danny's strength increased. He could rub his hands together for a few minutes, succeeding in making them warm.

Miriam had told me that a person should not remain passive when receiving a massage; otherwise, that person is receiving stimulation but not distributing or releasing the energy. During our third session, I asked Danny to do some simple motions while I worked on him, such as moving his head from side to side or bending and straightening his knee.

Danny's abdomen was tense and hard. I taught him to breathe through his nose, and this helped expand and relax his abdominal muscles and diaphragm. But his legs needed the most work, particularly the stronger leg; its contracted muscles were as hard as a rock. It took several months before Danny's legs could relax, but when this happened his whole body began to relax. His breathing, which had been extremely shallow, gradually deepened.

Then I began to massage Danny's head. It wasn't easy, because at first he couldn't bear to be touched there. When he was seven years old, he'd lost the hearing in one ear following an auto collision, and shortly after that the muscular dystrophy symptoms began to appear. It amazed me that his doctors didn't see the collision as a factor in his disease.

Whatever the cause, Danny's disease first appeared at age seven. It seemed to stop for a time while Danny was growing rapidly, but during his adolescence the deterioration process became obvious. By the time he was seventeen, when I met him, Danny had so much difficulty walking that he was almost ready for a wheelchair. After we came to know each other, he told me that he had decided to kill himself rather than ever use a wheelchair.

Danny was a special person, and a very troubled one. He told me that life was as meaningless as dust, and that he saw no reason to live. He was drawn to pessimistic philosophers like Sartre and Camus. For Danny, life was nothing but a prison, and death would be a release. But after we worked together for a few months, Danny began to see some results and his attitude improved remarkably. Suddenly he saw that there might be a way out. He looked upon his work with me as a possible reprieve. When he was able to walk a little more easily and lift his arms twice as high, he began to believe that there might be a chance of a cure.

Danny was disciplined in working on himself. He exercised for four hours every day. He developed his own system for working on himself: While watching TV or listening to music, he did very simple movements for up to half an hour each. He worked on his hands, arms, shoulders, legs, stomach, and chest, and he massaged everywhere he could reach. After three months, Danny decided to stop working with me and to continue by himself. For the next nine months, he worked alone and refused to see me. He considered working on his body as a kind of sculpting exercise, and he didn't want to show it to me until he was satisfied with the results. We stayed in touch during this time, but it was a while before I actually saw him again.

More Success with Muscular Dystrophy

MY NEXT MUSCULAR DYSTROPHY patient was Yankel, a goldsmith by profession. One day my grandfather dropped by my family's apartment to tell me that he had recommended me to a "one-legged man who wanted a massage." He added that it was lucky for me that the man had just one leg, because I'd only need to do half the work. He thought this was quite funny. I said, "If this man is one-legged, he needs more than a massage; he will need some specialized treatment." Grandfather answered irritably, "Are you telling me how to do massage?" (He knew nothing about massage, but assumed that since he was older he must know more about everything.) "Well, since you're such an expert," I teased, "why aren't you teaching the massage class I'm attending?" "It would take fifty years for you to learn what I know," he responded. "Here is his phone number. Don't forget to use talcum powder."

Yankel called me a few days later. He told me that he had progressive muscular dystrophy, and I agreed to come to his house. When I arrived, his wife told me, "There is no medical treatment that can help Yankel, but we are willing to try anything." Then Yankel entered the room with braces on both legs and supported by two canes. Though his legs were extremely thin, he was not "one-legged" as Grandfather had said. And as a result of his sedentary life, those thin legs had to support a rotund upper body.

I immediately began to work on Yankel's legs, and the massage gave him immense relief. His breathing became easier. His legs and feet, which were cold and stiff, now felt warm and relaxed. After I finished, Yankel wrote out a generous check without even asking what I charged. His appreciation of my work really bolstered my confidence.

Yankel was eager to continue treatment with me, and soon I became a regular visitor at his home. Yankel and his wife were warm Romanian people; they generously welcomed me as a member of their family.

I showed Yankel gentle exercises for his legs, and advised him to keep them in motion as much as possible, as his job was sedentary. Since his calves were very thin, I advised him to move his feet in a rotating motion to build up the calf muscles, then visualize that motion for a period of time, then rotate his feet again. I instructed him to make very small movements with his toes all day to strengthen his foot and calf muscles. It was hard for him to fully bend his knees, so I told him to lie on his back and turn his feet from side to side, increasing the circulation and building up the calf muscles. After eight sessions, he was able to bend his knees.

Next, I had Yankel lie on his back on a blanket with his feet on the floor, bend his knees, and make circles on the floor with his feet, moving the knees indirectly. I massaged him gently and rapidly to increase circulation as he did this. Another technique was to place my fingertips on a muscle and shake my hands so rapidly that the muscle vibrated, which created the feeling of electricity. Yankel improved rapidly, showing unmistakable gains in the strength and size of his leg muscles. His feet became more mobile and limber, and his balance while standing improved. After two months, he began to walk without the leg braces, and then he decided to give up one of the canes.

In fact, Yankel's improvement was so great that he became overconfident. One day as he was walking down the stairs, he threw one leg out to the side, the way he'd had to when he walked with braces on. The fragile leg slammed against the wall and, without the iron brace to protect it, broke easily. This was partly my fault; I had appreciated his eagerness to improve, knowing how badly I wanted to get rid of my glasses, but I hadn't realized how ingrained his old walking habits were. I had shown him how to walk properly, lifting each foot and carefully placing it down, but since he still had the habit of throwing his leg out to the side, he ended up in a cast.

Yankel wore the cast for six weeks, and I worked on him often during this time. He was always happy to see me. After the leg recovered, Yankel wore his braces for a while, then gave them up again. Though he found it difficult to walk properly, he did pretty well...until one day when, while exercising holding onto a chair, he started showing off for his wife. He pretended to kick her, and he lost his balance, fell down, and broke his leg again! This time his leg was in a cast for three months.

In spite of these setbacks, Yankel continued to bounce back. He enjoyed doing the exercises, and they benefited him. His legs grew thicker and stronger. One day he said to me, "You know, Meir, you owe me some money." I became very nervous. "What did I do? What money?" I asked. "The money I keep paying my tailor to refit my pants," he said with a grin. Yankel had lost thirty or forty pounds from all the exercise. The weight loss was helpful for him, as it had been difficult for him to support his heavy upper body with such skinny legs. He had come down four sizes in four months!

I took Yankel walking on the beach a few times, and his strength and confidence increased. His enthusiasm turned out to be greater than his patience, and Yankel found it difficult to settle for gradual improvement. With two leg fractures and the prospect of slow progress, he lost interest in working on himself. I was sad about this, for I felt that Yankel could have recovered completely.

An Emerging Practice

ALTHOUGH I WAS FRUSTRATED about Eli and Yankel, I knew that each of them had taught me a lot about the nature of neuromuscular disease and the necessity of patience and perseverance. I was eighteen and just out of high school, and I had already had three muscular dystrophy patients. Friends and relatives began to tell others about my work, and suddenly I had something of a practice. More than twenty people were coming to me for massage, exercise, and treatments — with many varieties of muscular, spinal, and neurological problems. The more people I worked on, the more sensitive my touch became. Miriam had taught me that everyone is different and that I would have to intuitively adjust my touch and my exercises for each person; increasingly, I found that I could do this.

I had come to understand that a therapist should never press on the muscles to the point of extreme pain. Especially in seriously ill patients, this can damage the nervous system and sometimes the whole body. Touch must be pleasant, not painful. Pressure may be increased gradually, as a person is ready for it and able to take it. A therapist must have very sensitive hands to know which touch is called for in each situation. I felt grateful to have developed the sensitivity of my fingers through all those years of studying Braille.

There was no magic secret to my work. I wasn't some fantastic healer who suddenly had hands full of electricity and uncanny power. I had to work on myself constantly, and I needed to massage my hands often, particularly before working with patients. My hands, which had been weak, were growing stronger. But I sensed that I was beginning to develop something new — a unique approach to the body.

CHAPTER 5

VERED: LEARNING FROM POLIO

Because I was now working with patients, the issue of credentials arose. Several friends and family members told me that I could be jailed for "practicing medicine without a license." So the summer following high school, I began to look into schools of physical therapy. One admissions director told me that I couldn't study at his school because of my vision problems. Another was so outraged by the work I was already doing without a license that she wouldn't consider my application.

My sister, Bella, had been living in San Francisco for a couple of years, and she thought it might be easier for me to get accepted into a school in America. I liked her idea, but it was out of the question; we simply did not have the money.

One day my aunt Esther, uncle Moshe's widow, telephoned. She had been completely opposed to my work on my eyes, and then to my work with other people. But seeing my determination to continue, she offered to help me get a professional degree in physical therapy. It wasn't that she suddenly approved of my work; she just wanted me to become respectable. In the past, she had suggested that I become a professor of Biblical studies or literature, but I had refused. When she finally understood that I had chosen a different direction, she decided to help me pursue it — but on her terms.

"I can't afford to send you to the United States," she told me, "but you could go someplace closer, like Italy. If you can't study in Israel, you shouldn't waste your time here." I was grateful for her offer. Since she had vigorously opposed my work for more than a year, her about-face was especially welcome — even though I knew that her motivation was not a real interest in my work, but her desire to make me a "somebody." While I resented her motives, I felt that she was right: I should take the opportunity to study abroad. So I accepted her offer.

Trying to Enter a Professional School

I PREPARED TO LEAVE FOR ITALY. I studied Italian and registered with the Italian consulate. After four months of planning and a month's delay during the Yom Kippur War with Syria and Egypt, I set off for Italy. Twelve days later, I was home again.

It turned out that the school's acceptance conditions hadn't been made clear to me by the Italian consulate. There were 270 candidates for twenty openings, eleven of which were filled before I arrived. I also learned that a degree in an Italian physical therapy school would not be recognized outside of Italy.

I had left with the equivalent of $450 — a generous sum at the time — and I returned with more than half of it left. My family told me privately that I'd been foolish not to take the opportunity to travel around Europe and have a vacation. But I felt that I had gone with a serious purpose, and I really didn't want to spend my aunt's money on a vacation. The abrupt change of plans was somewhat disappointing, but I was happy to be home. There was much to do.

Aunt Esther began to urge me to pursue another direction. She again took up the idea that I should become a professor of literature or philosophy. I told her that this was of no interest to me at all, and that I had my own goals and was eager to pursue them. "You have no direction," she insisted. "What you are doing is a waste of time."

I finally told her that I would rather be a masseur in a sauna than give up my work. "That's disgraceful!" she shouted. "You talk like a low-class bum." I was amused that my aunt, a founder of the Israeli Socialist Workers' Party, was suddenly so class-conscious.

Nothing would change Aunt Esther's mind. Even Savta agreed with her: "Esther is absolutely right. You should study literature and stop trying to make a living scratching other people's backsides." I was deeply hurt that even she felt this way, but there was nothing I wanted to do more than what I was doing.

I had grown steadily more successful in my work, and I met more and more people who were interested in it. It was easy for this to happen in Israel, because we are a very communicative — should I say nosy? — people, always interested in what others are doing. It was mostly from my family that I got arguments.

In fact, I was quite pleased with the direction of my life. I even had a real girlfriend, a beautiful girl named Yaffa who listened to my problems with sympathy and love. Her compassion helped me carry on in spite of the stress. And my work itself continued to be a great source of satisfaction.

Miriam always did her best to help me. The period when she was avoiding me turned out to be brief. One day, she arranged for me to meet a licensed physical therapist who worked in a hospital; he suggested that I try to get into a school of physical therapy for the blind in England. This sounded like a good idea, but for now I wanted to stay in Israel.

In the fall of 1973, I enrolled at Bar Ilan, a religious university outside Tel Aviv. I wanted to get into the biology program, but all of the science departments were full by the time I registered, so I enrolled in the philosophy department. This, of course, pleased my family, and I was happy enough. I had always been interested in philosophy, particularly Jewish philosophy, and there was an excellent department at Bar Ilan. My plan was to enter the biology program as soon as there was an opening.

Working with Vered's Polio

ONE DAY AT BAR ILAN, a beautiful, black-haired Moroccan woman sat down beside me in the cafeteria, offered me a cookie and a cup of coffee, and quite forwardly asked, "What do you do besides study?" She told me that her name was Vered, and I told her a little about my work on my eyes and my work with patients. She asked me, "Do you think you can help me? I have polio." "Of course!" I told her. We agreed to meet at my house the following day.

Vered had had five operations on her affected leg. During one operation, a piece of cement was implanted in her big toe to keep it straight. Her thigh muscles were very thin, and the calf and buttock of her weak side were almost fleshless. This forced her to walk and stand with all of her weight on the other leg. Walking was so painful that she had to stop and rest every five or six steps.

Vered had frequent, paralyzing headaches that often kept her out of class. Boring lectures caused her great physical discomfort. She was also too shy to enter the lecture hall if she was even a few minutes late. She was a perfectionist in everything she did; if she couldn't do something perfectly, she would give up.

Vered's family was very poor, and she hated this. Her father was disabled, and neither of her parents worked, so the family lived on welfare. Vered herself earned a little money by working after school.

Because of her charm and intelligence, Vered made friends easily, but she always felt that she was deceiving people. Her relationships seemed wonderful at first, but then she would gradually close herself off. There was some fear in her that made it impossible to fully open up to others. Perhaps this was because of her illness or her poverty. Whatever it was, this complex and contradictory person was the most attractive woman I had ever met. She had a mysterious kind of beauty, with a smile like the Mona Lisa. She was especially pretty when she was in a good mood, but her moods were very changeable.

Vered was also the most intelligent person I had ever met. It wasn't just her extraordinary range of knowledge and nearly perfect memory, but she was also completely honest and open to new things. She listened well, and she always understood new ideas; she not only understood what was said, but what was behind the words. She was therefore reluctant to look too closely at herself, afraid of her own clear and uncompromising insight. She could appreciate the good things in her character, but she was often dismayed by her own behavior, and disturbed when she couldn't control it. She sometimes found life to be wondrous, but mostly exhausting and impossible.

Vered often spent whole days and nights in bed, paralyzed by pain, depression, and fatigue. Most people occasionally wake up tired, not wanting to face the day, but Vered felt that way most of the time. The more she stayed in bed doing nothing, the worse she felt about herself and the world.

And yet, with all her frustrations, Vered kept on making new friends and welcoming new experiences. She seemed to step forward into the world with great confidence, but beneath the surface, her spirit, like her body, was frail and uncertain.

When Vered came to my home for the first session, I began by testing her weak leg. She could not even tolerate my lightly touching her kneecap because of the pain from the surgery. At the slightest touch, she cried out. The leg was twisted to one side because the muscles were too weak to hold it straight. All the operations had been harmful to her. It made me want to cry to see this weak and wasted leg, destroyed by the knives of surgeons. Yet I knew that she could be helped tremendously and that we would have to begin by building up her weak leg. I showed her a couple of simple exercises, and we agreed to meet again.

I saw Vered several times at school before our next session. She asked whether I needed any help in reading. When I said yes, she willingly sat and read to me from my textbooks. Her voice was clear and lovely.

I took Vered to meet Miriam, who was also charmed by her. She showed Vered a Czechoslovakian book for dancers, illustrating correct and incorrect postures of standing, sitting, and walking, and demonstrated some exercises that she thought might help Vered. One was a belly-dancing technique that consisted of rotating the hips in isolation from the rest of the body. Miriam felt that Vered understood this work as few people could, and she appreciated our work together.

Vered was unbelievably sensitive to pain; even an affectionate squeeze of the hand could bring her to the point of tears. The pain in her leg was terrible. It hurt her when I worked on her, but she made a great effort to endure it. I used oil to decrease the friction, and I showed her how to breathe deeply, which helped her relax a little and thereby reduce the pain.

I asked Vered to swing her arms up and down rhythmically while slowly moving her head from side to side. This released the tension in her shoulders and neck that naturally accumulates in people who have difficulty walking. Then I had her move one foot at the same time. Her foot could move only slightly, but by the end of an hour her circulation was so much better that I could touch the scarred area of her knee without her feeling much pain. She told me that she felt as if she were waking up from a horrible dream. After several more sessions, Vered began to notice that my touch was only occasionally painful — and then only where the deepest incisions had been made. The tissue beneath those scars was still deeply damaged, and some of the bones had never healed.

Vered did her exercises with the kind of determination I'd previously seen only in Danny and myself. She had a natural kinesthetic awareness, unlike anyone else I had ever met. After only two sessions, she was already creating new exercises to complement the ones I was giving her.

As our work progressed, I began to massage Vered underwater in the bathtub. Warm water relaxes the muscles, and movement underwater is easier. Some of Vered's muscles that normally couldn't move at all could move in the water, where there is less gravitational resistance. After three months, she was able to bend and straighten her knees evenly in the water; in six months she could do this out of water.

When she walked, Vered's knee tended to slip backward and lock, holding the leg rigid. This put a lot of pressure on her knee, jarring it with every step. This phenomenon was caused by the weakness of the muscles around the knee, and Vered and I concentrated on strengthening those muscles. One exercise she did for hours was to lie on her stomach and slowly raise and lower the calf of her weak leg. She then progressed to rotating the calf, slowly and gently working all the muscles around the knee. From being scarcely able to lift the leg at all, Vered increased the range of the movement until she could touch her buttock with her foot.

She also began to do self-massage, especially on her knee. Miriam always told me that, before doing massage, it is best to rub one's hands together until they are warm, and that the best way to do this is with the fingers interlocked while rubbing the palms together in a rotating motion. With her hands thus warmed, Vered would massage her knees. She did this almost constantly.

Vered especially loved the belly-dancing exercise. Her pelvic muscles were painfully contracted, and one hip was higher than the other; this exercise gently loosened her pelvis and hips. Her pelvic tightness came from the same source as most of her other problems: the imbalance in her movement caused by the weak leg. This imbalance caused some muscles to be overworked and strained, and others to be neglected and atrophied. The goal of her treatment was to create equilibrium. This was quite a job, since one leg was less than half the thickness of the other, all the way up to the hip.

Although polio is a rare disease these days, looking at the problems of a polio victim can teach us about other diseases as well. Orthopedic surgeons regard polio as a mechanical problem, as if these patients were malfunctioning machines. They cut into muscles, lengthening some and shortening others, breaking bones, moving bits of bone from one limb to another. In polio cases, the muscles being operated on are weak and atrophied; they do not have adequate nerve function or blood circulation. Surgery only further decreases their ability to function.

Many physical therapists try to activate a polio patient's muscles, but they don't emphasize balanced movement. Patients are told to bicycle or swim or do some other "therapeutic" exercise, but nothing is done to change their habitual ways of moving and using their bodies, their breathing, or their mental conceptions about movement. Instead of suggesting fundamental changes, physical therapists often try to help their patients improve by prescribing strenuous activities. They encourage heavy use of already strong limbs, rather than trying to strengthen the weak ones, for the simple reason that they don't think it's possible to strengthen the weak limbs. This is similar to the way my teachers wanted me to neglect my eyes. Today, we are seeing the results of this imbalanced approach in the form of heart attacks and strokes among polio patients — a result of what doctors call "post-polio syndrome." This condition seems to be caused by overexertion of one part of a polio patient's body — an arm or a leg — during the course of therapy or exercise.

Vered and I were trying to change the entire way her body worked — to build up muscles that had partially atrophied, and to encourage hitherto unused muscles to do the work of the degenerated muscles. We tried to balance her movement so that her two legs could work together, equally and in coordination.

Vered worked on this with both physical exercises and mental awareness. Each time she released part of her body from its habitual tension, she realized that she could, indeed, change her condition for the better. This experience transformed her attitude toward herself and her disease. *A small shift in attitude can make the difference between improvement and deterioration.*

Vered's exceptional intelligence and her ability to assimilate new ideas were assets in her therapy. She was always creating new exercises for herself, which I was then able to use with other patients with excellent results. I would ask her to visualize her weak leg being strong and healthy, and to picture herself walking as though she had two normal legs. The results were astounding. The difference in size between her two legs visibly decreased. Like almost everyone with weak legs, Vered had always tensed her arms and shoulders when she walked. But through breathing and slow leg exercises, alternating the two legs so that neither would become tired, she released much of this tension.

Vered and I often went to the beach to exercise, first walking in shallow water to accustom her to the movement of the waves, then wading in up to our waists. There she would stand, lifting one knee at a time to hip level. Out of the water, she could barely lift her leg at all, but in the water it was easy. This trained her weaker leg to lift itself with its own muscles, and it helped break her habit of dragging it along when walking on land. The muscles were there; they just needed the right conditions in order to develop.

When I first met Vered, she needed to rest every five or six steps when she walked. But with exercise, her strength increased to the point where she could walk as much as three miles without discomfort. She had to work up to this distance gradually, and her muscles ached as she increased the distance. But she learned to relieve the pain and fatigue through gentle stretching exercises and massage. Her improvement was nothing short of phenomenal.

Channi: Another Person with Polio

VERED INTRODUCED ME to her friend Channi, who also had polio. Channi had already consulted a number of "healers," and wanted nothing more to do with them. But Vered convinced her that I was not a "healer," but a teacher of movement, so she agreed to meet with me. Like Vered, Channi had been stricken with polio as an infant. Her right leg was the stronger one; she called it "my beautiful leg." Her left leg was as rigid and thin as a stick; she called it "my interesting leg." The "interesting" leg had survived nine operations. Her ankle had become so weak that, to prevent the foot from hanging loosely, the surgeons had installed a piece of her hipbone in it. This enabled her to walk without a leg brace, but she could not bend her ankle or move her foot.

Channi was attractive, but the damage to her leg had injured her self-esteem. She walked with a cane, and — as if the cane made it impossible for her to be pretty — she was careless about her grooming and dress.

Like Vered, Channi's weak leg was extremely sensitive to pain. In order for her to tolerate more than a half-minute massage on that leg, I had to constantly change the kind of touch I used, sometimes tapping, sometimes stroking, sometimes pinching lightly and quickly, always modulating the firmness of the touch. As her tolerance for this increased, the massage brought more circulation to the injured areas, helping them feel more alive.

Channi's leg had a tendency to become hot, especially when she walked too far or sat in an awkward position. Most polio patients have legs that feel cold to the touch, due to lack of circulation. In her case, however, tension caused the blood to flow to the surface, keeping it from reaching the deeper tissues. I massaged her leg gently with a vibrating motion, as I had with Yankel, and the accumulated fluid that had caused her leg to overheat slowly dispersed. Massage can regulate body temperature whether the body is overheated or chilled, since either can be caused by poor circulation. Channi learned to do this for herself, and it was her first success in the therapy. Although she had been skeptical, once she began to see some improvement, she was eager to continue with treatment. As she spent more time working on herself, I noticed that she also took better care of her appearance.

Channi and I frequently went to the beach to exercise. This would have been healthy for her even if only for the sunshine and the cleansing sea air, but my main purpose was to help her adapt to different walking conditions. I wanted her to learn to walk in sand, where the foot sinks in with each step and one must lift one's leg to pull it out. Polio patients typically drag their legs from the hips, rather than lifting them off the ground, so learning to walk on sand is very helpful. It was also helpful for Channi to learn to walk in the waves near the shore and to do leg exercises in the water, either sitting in shallow water or standing with my assistance. It is a challenge for any polio patient to keep balanced and upright while standing in the surf.

Channi found it difficult to walk in the sand; she lost her balance and tipped with each step. It was the same in the water: A wave that wouldn't affect a toddler would knock her over. So we approached these goals gradually, step-by-step. I gave her breathing exercises, massaged her legs before and after she tried to walk, and had her "walk" in the sand on her knees. I even stretched her legs by dragging her along the beach by her feet.

Little by little, Channi's balance and strength improved. After about a dozen sessions at the beach, she could stand upright in the water and walk in the sand for ten yards without falling. As a result, she could walk much better on solid ground with her cane, even though her foot was still immobile.

Channi's greatest improvement was in her thighs. I taught her to kneel with her heels under her buttocks, then separate her legs and sit on the floor between her heels. From there she would rise up onto her knees, then lower herself again. This forced her to use both thighs equally. In ordinary movement, she had hardly moved the thigh of her weaker leg at all.

The most effective exercise for Channi by far was a mental one. To help her develop movement in her affected ankle, which had been completely immobile since her doctors inserted the piece of bone to straighten it, I told her to rotate her stronger ankle and, at the same time, visualize the other ankle rotating. When she first tried this, she told me that she felt pain in the paralyzed ankle, as if it were actually moving. I told her that this was a good sign, and to continue the exercise. After six months of faithful practice, Channi did develop limited mobility in her ankle. It was then that she gave up her cane for many years afterward.

Many years later, I returned to Israel to give a workshop. Channi came to the workshop, and told me with pride that her cane had been sitting in the closet unused for more than ten years.

Frieda's More Severe Polio

I SOON BEGAN WORKING with a third young woman who had polio. Frieda's condition was even more severe than Channi's or Vered's. Both of her legs were paralyzed, and her abdominal muscles were extremely contracted from having to do the work of the legs. She suffered from chronic digestive disorders, as do many polio patients, because of cramped and imbalanced abdominal muscles.

Frieda also had a serious back problem. Early in her childhood, her doctors had noticed that she was unable to hold her back straight. They were concerned about the possibility of progressive degeneration of the spine, so they implanted a platinum rod in her back. She had braces on both legs and on her neck. When I tested her, I discovered that one foot seemed to have some potential for movement, and that the knee of the same leg could also move slightly. I thought that this could develop later into enough of a motion to activate and strengthen the leg and eventually eliminate the need for a brace.

With my therapy, Frieda improved to the point where she could move her foot a little. Then, just as she was developing some movement in the stronger leg, she stopped coming to me. Instead, she began to see a

Feldenkrais therapist, who concentrated on improving her back muscles so that she would be more comfortable. He didn't even try to improve her legs. I have seen this again and again: Someone who experiences a little improvement becomes frightened and withdraws from the therapy.

Learning as I Went Along

THERE CAME A TIME when I no longer needed to search for new exercises for myself or others; they would just come to me when I needed them. While working on myself, I would meditate on what I was trying to accomplish, and inspiration for new exercises would come — exactly the right exercises for my back, my legs, my eyes. This also began to happen in regard to my patients; by attuning myself to them and their needs, I knew what to do with them.

The needs of handicapped people are basically the same as those of anyone else. We must activate parts of the body that are dormant and unused, and strengthen the rest of the body in order to create proper, balanced functioning. When handicapped people start to work on themselves, their movements are often abrupt, strained, and insensitive. When they massage themselves, they are usually rough at first. It is especially helpful for handicapped people to learn to massage others before trying to massage themselves. After learning to be sensitive and caring toward another person's body, it is easier to extend the same consideration toward oneself. This is especially true of handicapped people, who often feel hatred toward their own bodies.

I learned a great deal about working with the handicapped from Vered, Channi, and Frieda. Most people do not use their bodies properly and have a strong resistance to learning how to do so. This is especially pronounced in the case of the handicapped. They try to separate themselves from the crippled part of the body, so it is hard for them to work on those areas.

My task was to try to help my handicapped patients come into touch with bodies from which they had become alienated. I was trying to help them regenerate functions that they had given up hope of ever regaining — or even to gain functions they'd never had before. I was discovering something about the psychology of illness, along with its physiology. I learned that a person must be willing to recover in order to overcome limitations.

CHAPTER 6
OUR FIRST CENTER

My practice continued to grow. One of my patients, Lyuba, was acquainted with the director of the Vegetarian Society, the main organization of alternative and complementary medicine in Israel. Lyuba told the director about me, and he invited me to give a lecture there.

I was thrilled! I hadn't lectured before, and I looked forward to speaking publicly about what I'd been doing. But the prospect of my first lecture was short-lived. When I met with the society's director to make the arrangements, he discovered that I was not a vegetarian myself, so he withdrew the invitation and suggested that, instead, I meet with several of the physicians at the society's clinic.

That was how I met Dr. Frumer. Dr. Frumer had suffered two heart attacks, and subsequently realized that he had to change his ways to prevent another. He underwent a twenty-day fast, and this lowered his blood pressure and normalized his weight. After that, he began exercising twenty minutes each day, eating a balanced vegetarian diet, and leading a less stressful life. His improvement was immediate, and he became a staunch advocate of exercise and good nutrition.

This change was not well received by either Dr. Frumer's patients or his superiors, who preferred the usual alleviation of symptoms by drugs and surgery. A few of his patients welcomed the new methods and actually wanted to change their lifestyles, and his methods worked for them. Most of them, however, were angry and upset with the suggested changes. They either didn't want to change, or they were convinced that drugs had to be the most effective treatment. They complained to the village clinic where Dr. Frumer worked about his unorthodox methods (juice diets, fasting instead of antibiotics to reduce fever, and so on). His superiors listened to these complaints, but they turned a deaf ear to his success stories — even a case of gangrene that he had successfully treated through fasting. They simply told him that he could follow standard medical practice, or leave.

Dr. Frumer resigned from his practice and came to the Vegetarian Society. There he found a niche for himself, primarily as an advocate of a well-known reducing diet for overweight women. His new practice wasn't large, but he enjoyed the pressure-free environment in which he could use simple, natural methods to work with his patients. When I met Dr. Frumer, he was enthusiastic about what I had to say, and I even interested him in working on his own eyes. He eventually persuaded the Vegetarian Society to allow me to lecture and to see patients at their clinic.

The Birth of a New Therapy Center

AROUND THE SAME TIME, Vered and I decided to start a center where we could see patients and teach the therapeutic techniques we were developing. Vered had a gift for this work, and she had begun helping me with some of my patients. We also decided to invite Danny to work with us. Although Danny was working on himself independently of me, we were still in touch. I would see him once a week for the best massage I've ever received. Muscular dystrophy patients are expected to degenerate, but Danny was actually improving. He could now not only lift his arms normally, but he was even lifting light weights. He could climb stairs well, and his fingers had built up from being pencil-thin to being thick and strong, with incredible energy and sensitivity. I knew he would be an asset to our center.

As you can imagine, the prospect of having such a place aroused nearly uncontrollable enthusiasm in me. Not only could we work with patients, but we could work on each other, help each other with patients, and learn together. But when I talked about this with Danny, he was reluctant to join us. He didn't think he could communicate well enough in his limited Hebrew, and he didn't feel qualified to work with patients. I reminded him that he had the best touch of anyone I knew, including Miriam, and told him to just look at his own body if he needed proof of his abilities. He finally agreed.

We found an apartment near Dizengoff Street, one of the main business, shopping, and entertainment areas of Tel Aviv. We had planned to simply start a center for bodywork, but it soon became clear that this was also a good place for us to live. Vered had her own room, and Danny and I shared one large room. It took me a while to earn the money to buy a sliding door to divide the room; until we installed it, Danny and I had little privacy. Vered's room was across the corridor. None of us had ever lived away from home before, and this "center" provided everything we wanted: rooms to work in, our own kitchen, and two large verandas, open to the sun, which Vered filled with potted flowers and plants. The atmosphere was warm and homelike.

Vered and I worked on patients on mattresses on the floor, and I bought a massage table for Danny because it was difficult for him to sit on the floor. The table creaked and wobbled, but it worked, and the three of us were in heaven.

My family had become resigned to my career choice, and they supported my new business by sending people to us. In addition to the patients who were referred by my family, our friends, and other patients, the Vegetarian Society clinic had signed up several patients to work with me there. Of these, only two actually kept their appointments, but one of them — an older woman who talked nonstop — got many others interested in our therapy.

I liked working at the Vegetarian Society clinic. I was associated with licensed physicians, and they referred patients to me. This was not only flattering, it meant that I was under their protection and had the support of the 2,000-member society. After only a few weeks there, I had a full schedule of patients.

When I finally gave my first lecture at the Vegetarian Society, about 150 people showed up, and they were very attentive. I talked about my work with my own eyes, and about the work of Dr. Bates. Afterward, audience members asked many questions. Although there were a few objections to specific things I had said, such as my blanket disapproval of sunglasses (which I will explain in chapter 8), on the whole the lecture was well received. I began to have even more requests for appointments.

Working with Eye Problems

MANY OF MY EARLY PATIENTS had eye problems. One of the first, Mr. Vardi, had cataracts on both eyes, one of which was so mature that his lens was almost completely opaque. He could see only a little light and shadow. I doubted that his poorer eye could be helped, but I gave him some exercises for his better eye. I showed him the five basic eye exercises: palming, sunning, shifting, blinking, and swinging.

Eye Exercise: Swinging

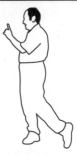

In swinging, you stand in one place, hold one finger in front of your face one or two feet away from you, and then turn the body from side to side while looking at the finger. You pivot on the ball of the foot, and see the visual field as moving in the opposite direction. Doing this exercise increases detail vision and makes shifting automatic.

After four months, Mr. Vardi could see his fingers with his bad eye — a great improvement for him. I tried to help him further by showing him the correct way to read. Most people read a word or a sentence, or even an entire line, at a time. In order to make the best use of our eyes, we must see just one point at a time. Instead of taking in larger units, such as lines or sentences, we should read word by word, letter by letter, and then point by point.

Good vision consists of seeing central details vividly and the periphery less clearly. The center point of the retina, which is called the macula, is the part of the eye that sees with the greatest acuity, but it can only see a small portion of the visual field at a time. Therefore, in order to fully use the macula, we must constantly shift our point of focus from one small detail to the next. Eyes that see well do this automatically and unconsciously. Eyes that see poorly must consciously relearn the habit of "shifting," for they have formed the habit of staring fixedly and straining to take in the entire visual field at once, whereby the use of the macula is lost, making clear vision impossible.

This is especially true in reading, where the greedy mind grabs for whole sentences at a time, straining the eyes to see in a way for which they were not designed. This can damage the eyes permanently, even causing cataracts. Reading point by point is different from the way most people are taught, but it is how the eyes work naturally.

It was a real challenge for Mr. Vardi to distinguish between letters, or even between words; over many years, he had developed the habit of reading an entire line at a time. Although his cataracts didn't disappear, by practicing these exercises he was able to avoid surgery, and his vision improved considerably.

An elderly woman named Tovah also came to see me; she'd had three operations for cataracts, a detached retina, and glaucoma. She was almost totally blind; all she could see was a little sunlight. "Sometimes people come to me too late," I told the secretary of the Vegetarian Society. I will never forget his answer: "People come to you the way they are, and that's where you start." Tovah did, in fact, begin to experience some improvement after working on her eyes. One day, while sitting in front of the post office, she was able to see people coming and going. It was only temporary, but similar flashes of sight began to occur, and she was quite encouraged.

Tovah brought her granddaughter, Mazel, who had vision problems, too. Mazel not only learned the exercises, but also took an interest in the theory behind them. She began to observe carefully how her own eyes worked and how they reacted in various situations. She felt in herself a resistance to seeing clearly, something many people with sight problems experience. Mazel realized that her extreme sensitivity to light and to such substances as chlorinated swimming pool water was caused by a general anxiety about her environment. As she learned to relax her eyes, Mazel began to take pleasure in seeing. She began psychotherapy, and was able to use her eyes to become more comfortable with herself and her surroundings.

Different Therapeutic Styles

DANNY, VERED, AND I had different insights based on our individual experiences of curing ourselves of muscular dystrophy, polio, and blindness. Together, we were able to help a wide range of patients.

Danny had an acute sense of how muscles became tight and how to release them. He usually worked directly on a patient's tightest area, slowly releasing the tension until the tissues were softened and relaxed. Even though he only worked on a few contracted muscles, the patient's whole body would be much more relaxed. I never worked this way; a patient's tightest area was the last thing I would touch. I worked, instead, on all the related points. For example, for a person with a headache, I worked on the neck, shoulders, back, and stomach before even touching the head.

Danny's exercises were also much simpler and more direct than mine. Working on himself, he followed the same routine every day. He found it most important that an exercise have a direct relationship to the problem. He had to see that an exercise either built up a muscle or released it from tension. Again, my approach was different. I was most interested in the interrelationships among different parts of the body. I tried to activate the whole body, bringing the patient into an entirely different state of being. My movements were directed toward changing the entire rhythm of the body.

Vered leaned toward my way of working, but both she and Danny were finding techniques best suited to themselves. Just as a patient must develop a unique approach in order to really improve, a therapist must find a unique way to help each patient. One's experiences with working on one's own body often determine the way one works on others.

Danny, Vered, and I were developing a working relationship and a great feeling of camaraderie. We often exercised together, then shared our discoveries and experiences. It was as if we shared a meditation of body and spirit. It was the deep bond of three handicapped people who had made a decision to overcome their handicaps and were working together to achieve that goal. We shared a truth that surmounted the ignorance and prejudices of the world around us. Our center was a warm, protecting place where we could be ourselves without fear.

This camaraderie was not confined to us. People loved to visit our center. There were some patients who, as Vered said, stuck to our center like chewing gum. People sensed the atmosphere of security, reassurance, and optimism that arose from our conviction that we, ourselves, would get better. We all knew that my vision would continue to improve, that Vered's leg would grow stronger, and that Danny would completely recover.

Fortunately, when we started our center we already had a physician's approval and support. Dr. Frumer of the Vegetarian Society was always on our side. He referred many patients to us, and he made sure that they were patients we could safely work on. If he thought that a patient's condition might deteriorate in spite of our good work, he would not refer them to us, just to be sure that we had no legal difficulties.

Danny, Vered, and I realized that the natural state of the body is health. We shared this understanding with the Vegetarian Society, where the doctors felt that the causes of illness can always be found, although they believed that diet was usually the main factor. We agreed with them that a poor diet has harmful effects and a good diet is beneficial, but we found that the way you move and the way you breathe are more important. We came to know that, once the body was relaxed, the breathing correct, and all the joints completely flexible, it was difficult for any disease to take hold.

Learning to Relate with Patients

OFTEN DANNY, VERED, or both of them, joined me in my work at the Vegetarian Society. We had many kinds of patients, mostly with minor problems. Many were elderly, and their problems stemmed from years of misusing their bodies. Most of them didn't come to us with the idea of learning to heal themselves; they simply wanted to be "treated," massaged, or just given a little attention. They seldom exercised at home, and they seemed content with the temporary relief they received during a session. As members of the Vegetarian Society, they already had some sound ideas about health, and they could appreciate our work and utilize it somewhat, even if not to its full extent.

A few of our patients were true hypochondriacs who actually did not want to be cured. They came to give our work a try and, after a couple of sessions with their ailments safely intact, they felt satisfied that they had tried the latest treatment and it, too, couldn't help them.

We gave our full attention to each patient, no matter how much or how little he or she appeared to respond. We always explained to patients what we were doing and how they could help themselves. It was clear to me that no time spent on anyone was ever wasted. Our instincts and intuitions about people became sharper, and we quickly came to recognize the kind of people for whom this work is especially rewarding. I even began to dream about founding a hospital where patients would be treated with these self-healing methods we were using, and a school where practitioners could be trained in self-healing.

By this time, we already had a sizable following. Our practice continued to grow as a result of my lectures and the publicity the Vegetarian Society gave us, together with the recognition and referrals of several other physicians. We began to understand and demonstrate most of the fundamentals about illness and cures that became the basis of the Self-Healing Method. We realized the importance of meditating on the cures of our patients. Miriam used to tell me that I needed to think for hours before each session about the person I would treat, and I found this essential. Danny, Vered, and I found that our hands often knew much better than our heads what was best in a particular treatment.

Whenever someone initially came to us, I would test the patient first, followed by Danny and Vered. Usually Vered's prognosis was the most pessimistic, and Danny's the most optimistic. We never refused a patient on the grounds that we couldn't be of help; Danny felt that anyone could be cured from any disease.

Once, long before, when I had taken a friend with me to visit Uncle Moshe in the hospital, my friend said to me, "No matter how rich, wise, famous, or clever you are, you always end up here." This is often true, but I would now like to add: No matter how badly off you may be, or how handicapped, there is a strong power within you that can always heal you or, at least, make your situation better. No matter how isolated you feel, your higher self is always there to be your best friend. Knowing this, you needn't feel isolated, fearful, or helpless. Our power of healing exists in every muscle of our bodies, every brain cell, every nerve fiber, every blood vessel. We are born with the power to heal ourselves, and we only need to rediscover it. Finding this power is like opening a closet and locating what you've been looking for everywhere. It was there all the time, but you just didn't see it. We search everywhere for cures for our diseases, not realizing that there is a force within us that has an infinite capacity to heal the body. This capacity is far more powerful than any disease. Disease exists only when we overlook this healing power.

Contrary to the common understanding of disease as something bad, we discovered that disease has a positive side. Disease is an indicator of a person's state of being, and the symptoms are a clear statement about how that person uses his or her body. We found, for example, that patients with cataracts had probably used their eyes rigidly for years, tensing them, staring with them, and not blinking enough. Our job was to help them become aware of the habits that created and were creating the condition, and to help them learn better habits. This was necessary in order for a real cure to come about.

In modern life, most of our activities are tightly scheduled. We seldom have time to relax and pay attention to how we feel and what our bodies need. Like a child, the body demands attention — and even more so when we try to ignore it. By becoming sick or disabled, the body forces us to listen.

Most people are quite passive about disease. Modern medicine encourages us to be preoccupied with the treatment of symptoms and to allow our bodies to be manipulated like machines. It is too obvious and too frightening to look carefully and try to discover the source of the problem. An obvious example is the emphysema patient who continues to smoke.

Shlomo, the elderly man who taught me exercises at the beach, understood the importance of giving the body a lot of loving attention. He worked on himself for two hours every day. Some people who came to our center were able to comprehend that every disease has its own cause and its own cure — that there was a reason for their problems, a cause for their symptoms, and a way to resolve these problems. These people would work with us until they knew exactly how to work on themselves; they learned what we showed them, and they learned to make their own discoveries about their bodies and minds and about what would help them. Such people always found the best ways to work on themselves. Every person who suffers from a disease must discover how to get at the cause, then learn how to find a cure. This process is difficult — and infinitely rewarding.

Internal Resistance to Healing

VERED IS A GOOD EXAMPLE of both the difficulty and rewards of this process. I taught her to use her weaker leg instead of overprotecting it — to lift it instead of dragging it. It was extremely difficult for her to do this. In order to succeed, she needed a strong inner voice to constantly remind her of her goals. Even after she realized that she was walking incorrectly, her resistance to change was deep. When her walking finally showed some improvement, I instructed her to climb stairs using both legs equally. This was nearly impossible at first, since her right leg was almost paralyzed, but she learned to do it. She also learned to walk on sand, which required bringing new muscles into play. With all of these exercises, Vered's progress was enormous. Yet when she was at the point where she could have completely overcome her limp, she hesitated. Her limp had become an integral part of her identity, and it was difficult to abandon it. I think that Vered was more aware of her true feelings than most people. None of us want to give up accustomed behavior. It is difficult to be aware of these ingrained attitudes that often run counter to reason and good judgment.

Another example was a patient of ours named Reuven, who had poor blood circulation to his feet and head. When he came to us, his face was bluish; because of impaired circulation, one cheek was partly paralyzed. He also had difficulty breathing and had occasional asthma attacks and digestive problems, but his fundamental problem was a bad self-image.

Reuven was only twenty-eight years old, but he felt defeated, having been in and out of hospitals for most of his adult life without a definite diagnosis. He had tried a number of diets and therapies. During our first session with Reuven, his face took on a normal pinkish color from the massage and exercises we did. He began to come to us regularly, and he seemed to enjoy the sessions. After only a few months, he was on the verge of a complete recovery; his cheek was no longer paralyzed, his circulation was greatly improved, his breathing was free and relaxed, and the circulation to his feet was quite normal. Then he stopped coming to our center. Sometimes, at this crucial point, the patient's unconscious resistance to new patterns keeps him from making the final step toward healing or success. Reuven discovered that old X-rays showed that he had a hole in one lung. Even though this in no way needed to prevent his full recovery, he suddenly told us that his condition was incurable and nothing could remedy it.

The Power of the Mind

AT ABOUT THIS TIME, I began to observe the importance of the mind in healing the body. I had been slowly raising and lowering my arm, trying to relax and breathe deeply. Then I realized that I was not paying attention to the movement of the arm or to the arm's sensations. I raised my arm again, and this time I noticed that it felt heavy and tense. I did this a few more times, and it still felt heavy. So I stopped for a while and simply visualized myself raising my arm. To my surprise, I found that the arm felt tense and heavy even in my imagination! I continued to visualize the movement until I could imagine the arm feeling light and the movement feeling easy. Then I tried the movement again, and the arm actually felt a lot lighter and moved much more easily.

I was excited about this discovery. I practiced with this technique for a long time, visualizing the arm as light, then as heavy, and found that I could influence my actual movement quite a lot. I immediately realized the implications that this had for my work with patients. I saw that the mind can help achieve relaxed, effortless motions, and that it is possible to bring about great changes in body functioning, just through awareness.

CHAPTER 7
BRACES FOR RIVKA

A little while before we opened our center, Miriam had referred a girl named Rivka to Vered and me. Rivka was nine years old and had been confined to a wheelchair with polio since the age of two. She had been fitted with leg braces three times, but because she was unable to straighten her left knee, her walking placed so much pressure on the braces that they always broke.

Vered and I went to Rivka's home together. It was on a side street in a crowded industrial area of Tel Aviv. A long flight of broken-down stairs led up to her family's apartment on the second floor. The small three-room dwelling housed eleven people; Rivka was the seventh of nine daughters. Her father had broken his back, disabling him permanently so that he couldn't work. Her mother didn't work outside the home either, so the family was mainly supported by the government, although some of the sisters worked. One sister was a nurse, another was a soldier, and the others were still in school. The apartment was dark and desolate inside. Rivka was sitting in her wheelchair and looking at the floor, her eyes hidden behind thick glasses. She was a shy little girl and very small for her age.

We tested Rivka's afflicted leg. Both of her legs were very thin, and they were expected to become paralyzed. Her back was stooped and had a lateral curvature in the middle of the spine. One of her arms was very weak; she could lift it chest-high only with a great deal of effort. The other arm was relatively normal. Her neck muscles were so weak that she could hardly hold her head up.

Vered and I tried to convince Rivka's sisters that she could be helped. I explained that the first thing she needed was massage to improve her circulation and bring warmth to her cold limbs; after that, some gentle movements could bring flexibility and strength. I showed them that she did have some capacity for movement, even in the semi-paralyzed leg, and that the movement in all the limbs could be improved. I emphasized, however, that improving her circulation was the first essential step. The sister who was a nurse tried to argue with me. In nursing school, she had learned that circulation could only be increased via nerve stimulation. She believed that Rivka's nervous system had been too badly damaged by the polio to provide the necessary circulation. I interrupted her, saying, "Yes, but blood flow can also increase nerve stimulation. Why don't you at least let her try our work?"

Then Vered quietly and confidently told Rivka's sisters about the progress that she had made with her own polio, first through working with me and then carrying on by herself. They agreed to try our therapy, with Vered acting as Rivka's chief therapist. Vered took the job with some reluctance; she was already working, carrying a full course-load at the university, dealing with her physical limitations, and working on her own legs. She was reluctant to add the long bus ride and walk twice a week to get to Rivka's apartment. At that point, Vered also wasn't fully confident of her abilities. But even with all her doubts and objections, she was excited at the prospect of treating a polio patient of her own, so she accepted the challenge.

Beginning to Work with Rivka

AT FIRST, RIVKA'S FAMILY OFFERED Vered little support in her efforts. The full extent of their cooperation was that one of the sisters tried to encourage Rivka to do the exercises Vered showed her. The little girl was not very cooperative at first, making it clear that she enjoyed her exercises about as much as most children enjoy homework. At first, Vered found working with Rivka frustrating. But after four visits, Rivka showed some motivation and changes began to take place. Her cold feet grew warm more rapidly with each treatment. She became more capable of limited movement. She could move her feet sideways, backward, and forward. Several of her arm and leg muscles grew stronger and appeared to be more developed. She could even lie on her back and raise her legs for several moments at a time.

Rivka's biggest problem was her difficulty in working on herself when Vered wasn't there. Rivka's home was small and crowded, offering little privacy or space in which to exercise. Vered worried that this might interfere with Rivka's growing enthusiasm. After talking it over, Vered and I decided that better surroundings were what Rivka needed most. At that point we had just opened our center, so we asked Rivka's family to bring her there for treatments. At first she was able to get a ride to the center, accompanied by one of her sisters, in the van that transported handicapped children to their special schools. After the treatment, we sent her home in a cab; we cut the already nominal cost of her sessions in half so that she could afford the cab fare. Then the van driver decided that our center was too far out of his way, and he refused to bring her there anymore. We had no alternative but to see Rivka at no charge so that she could afford to take a cab both ways.

In the beginning, most of the exercises we gave Rivka were to be done while she was lying face down on a mat. In this position, she would raise the foot of her stronger leg, then let it drop down onto her buttock. Then, with great effort from her back and stomach muscles, she raised the leg and returned it to the mat. This exercise was strenuous for her, and she could only accomplish it after repeated efforts, alternating with visualizing the foot moving up and down. But after a few weeks of practice, she could do it for five minutes at a time before she needed to rest. She would alternate exercise and rest, keeping this up for hours at a time.

The muscles in Rivka's legs were so contracted that her legs were always bent at the knees. We tried to straighten them by gently rotating them. Rivka also worked on her arms, first rotating her wrist, then with great effort doing the same with her elbow. It was most important for us to stimulate her sluggish circulation so that her nearly paralyzed body could enjoy at least the feeling of motion.

When Rivka came to our center, she stayed for several hours to work on herself. She sat on a couch on the veranda, and we often looked out the window to see how she was doing. She would sit there moving her neck, then her arms, then her hands, or she would lie on her stomach rotating her foot and breathing deeply. Often we would see her simply sitting with her eyes closed or staring up at the sky. When I asked her what she was doing, she would say, "I'm resting." I would give her five minutes to rest, then gently insist that she get back to work. She needed many such rest breaks. Nevertheless, she spent three to four hours working on herself each time she saw us. Danny was less patient and more insistent that she work hard, and she usually worked harder when he was watching.

A Stumbling Block

WHEN WE HAD BEEN WORKING with Rivka for three months, the three of us held a meeting to determine the next step in her treatment. We decided it was time for her to get braces again and begin to walk. She was suffering from lack of stimulation, both physical and mental; neither her home nor her school for the handicapped could provide that stimulation. Only at our center did she experience the freedom and activity she needed. We agreed that it was essential for her to become more mobile — that she needed to put more of herself into action. "We have to get her walking," Danny said. "If she doesn't walk, she is not going to use her muscles enough."

We talked with Rivka's family and suggested that they ask her school's orthopedist to order some braces for her. The orthopedist, however, refused to request government aid to pay for the braces. When I heard that, I decided to speak to him myself. I asked Rivka's sister Rachel, who had agreed that Rivka needed the braces, to accompany me and help me persuade him.

The orthopedist seemed a bit nervous, welcoming Rachel quite formally. Rachel introduced me as a good friend of the family. He invited us to sit down, and asked rather abruptly why we had come. When Rachel explained that we had come to repeat the family's request for braces, he became impatient. He told us that he had no intention of ordering braces for Rivka at that time because he planned to operate on her knee within six months, and she would need a different set of braces after the operation. He didn't want to waste taxpayers' money on two sets of braces.

I explained that Rivka was trying a new kind of therapy that might make such an operation unnecessary. I didn't introduce myself as the therapist, but I tried to describe the therapy itself. The orthopedist listened with surprising patience. He had expected nothing more than a routine request, which he would either grant or refuse. But as he listened, his interest grew and his abruptness disappeared. He was curious about our work — enough so that I decided to tell him I was Rivka's therapist. I told him about some of the movements we used to relax and strengthen her muscles, and he asked with a hint of sarcasm, "So what do you need the braces for?" I explained that she needed the braces for the greater mobility they would give her, to support her process of learning to walk.

He asked me, "What are you studying?" When I answered that I was studying philosophy, he demanded, "Then why do you want to argue about medicine? It is not your field. Leave the medical matters to me." "I'll be happy to leave medicine to you," I said, "but right now Rivka needs braces."

He gave me a kind, patient smile and said, "Look, young fellow, you are trying to do the impossible. Her knee cannot be straightened because her muscles are in constant spasm. She has broken her braces many times in the past because when she tries to walk, it puts more pressure on them than they can withstand, even though they are designed to support a much heavier person. There is only one solution to the problem: We will surgically break her knee in order to straighten the leg. Then she'll be able to use the braces without breaking them."

I asked him, "What if I can straighten the knee?" "There is no way in the world you can do that," he retorted, then added, "You know, I'm smarter than you think I am." He went on to tell me a number of stories to demonstrate his intelligence. "I never let anyone put anything over on me," he finished, "and I won't let you do it, either. But I'm willing to make a deal with you. I will recommend the braces; then you and I will make an agreement before a notary and a couple of witnesses that if you are not able to straighten her knee within six months, you will pay for the braces."

I was not intimidated. I thanked him and said I would think about it. "Take your time," he smiled. "I'll be happy to see you again if you decide to make the agreement."

Rachel and I left his office with mixed feelings. We had made some headway, but we knew it would be very hard to predict how long it would take us to straighten Rivka's leg. It might easily take longer than six months. The fact that the doctor had planned to perform his surgery at that time didn't guarantee that Rivka's leg could conform to his schedule. Straightening and strengthening her leg by our methods was bound to be a slow, painstaking process.

Most physical therapists would attempt to straighten Rivka's leg by stretching it forcefully. But her muscles were too tight to be stretched in that way. I was sure that the only way to straighten her leg was to relax the muscles and gradually strengthen them — and that the only way to achieve that was to keep the leg muscles working and moving. I felt that the motions used in walking would be especially effective. It was absolutely necessary that she get braces and begin to walk.

I told Rachel that, even if we didn't succeed in straightening Rivka's leg in half a year, at least Rivka would get her braces if we accepted the orthopedist's proposal. I was perfectly willing to take on the responsibility of paying for them if we failed. Rachel was deeply touched. Her sister Mazel, however, was not at all pleased; she insisted that the government should pay for the braces. As a nurse, she was accustomed to having the government supply everything a patient needed.

With or without the support of the orthopedist, Rivka, her sisters, and I were all convinced that the braces were essential. She needed movement, variety, a new environment, and an escape from the stifling atmosphere of her home and school. It was difficult and inconvenient for her to always be carried or pushed in a wheelchair. She had to have braces to achieve any degree of freedom.

I discussed the problem with my friends. One friend suggested that I ask the orthopedist for more time. I agreed with this, both because I doubted that six months would be enough time, and because I was afraid that the deadline might cause me to work too intensively with her, which would be hard on both of us. So I decided to ask the doctor to change his terms.

After two weeks, Rachel and I returned to the orthopedist's office. He welcomed me with a challenging grin and said, "So, what have you decided? Do we have a bet?" "Yes," I answered, "but I want you to give me two years." His jaw dropped in amazement, then outrage replaced his shock. "Get out of here, you charlatan," he said. That made Rachel angry, and she shouted at the orthopedist, "I don't want my sister to have that operation at all if you aren't going to help us now!" "I'm only trying to help Rivka," he answered patiently. "All I want is what's best for her." He turned back to me and asked, "What about eight months?"

"Forget it," I said. "We're not in a marketplace. If you give me two years, she is going to have a straight leg. I'm perfectly willing to bet, though, that in eight months she'll have a noticeably straighter leg."

"No," he replied. "I'm not going to make deals with a quack. I want a straight leg within six to eight months and, if not, you have to pay for the braces." At that point we left; it was clear that another solution had to be found.

I was in a state of shock. No one had ever called me a quack before, and I had been working on people for years. When Aunt Esther heard the story, she smiled and said, "Well, now you've learned your lesson. You'd better be prepared to hear the same thing from other people."

Rivka's doctor had refused to even consider that our work might have some validity. I felt that this was an insult, not only to me but to the truth. Many other doctors I had met would have done everything in their power to seek out any method that could have helped their patients. Even if he didn't have the imagination to understand the work in theory, the results would have spoken for themselves. I hadn't really expected him to go along with my plan, but I was nevertheless disappointed and rather depressed. I remained, to some degree, in a state of shock for a long time after that interview.

When I told Dr. Frumer what the orthopedist had said to me, he was amazed; he made it clear that he disagreed. It was a relief to know that I had the support of an established physician who understood and approved of what I was doing. I was unwilling to repeat the experience I'd had with Rivka's doctor, but as the shock wore off I regained my equilibrium. I wasn't afraid that the orthopedist would take legal action against me, even though he considered me a fraud. I realized that, while he doubted my abilities and rejected my proposal, he didn't actually oppose me. He simply couldn't support me.

That was when I realized that there is a big difference between "opposing" and "not accepting." When you cannot accept something, a part of you is aware, either consciously or subconsciously, that you are coming up against your own limitations. In the orthopedist's case, there was an element of fear involved. He was afraid to discover that something so contrary to his training, education, and beliefs might work — might be, indeed, exactly what his patients needed. He didn't want to challenge his training and past practice.

Even if the orthopedist had wanted to oppose me, he would have had no grounds for doing so; I could show results that proved the validity of my approach. But the doctor was unwilling to even investigate my work. If he had come to watch us work on Rivka — with gentle massage, circular movements of the joints, and slow, gradual stretching of her muscles — it might very well have changed his attitude.

The Kindness of Strangers

WE KNEW THAT we had to get braces for Rivka in one way or another. The question was: how? The solution came to us quite by surprise. At the time, Vered's friend Channi had a roommate named Tirza, who was the assistant producer of a weekly radio program. Tirza was interested in the work we were doing. When Tirza offered to interview us on the radio, it occurred to me that this might be an excellent way to solicit donations for Rivka's braces. I wanted to let the public know how important it was for us to help Rivka and others like her.

The time scheduled for the interview was ideal. It would run for fifty minutes on Friday evening — just after people returned home from work, and just before television programming for the evening began. The program was well publicized in the newspapers, and we had reason to believe that close to half a million people would hear it. The recording of the broadcast took between five and six hours, but when it was edited down to fifty minutes it was quite different than what we had expected; the interviewers had tried to sensationalize our work. Instead of the informal personal interview we had given them, they created a sort of official documentary.

Nevertheless, the program made a good enough impression to attract a lot of attention. We raised more than enough money to buy the braces for Rivka, and a good part of it came from Tirza herself. It was a wonderful boost to Rivka's therapy.

Dramatic Improvement

IN ORDER TO WALK with braces, Rivka would also need to use crutches, which required that she strengthen her arms. She had been practicing imagining her hands lifting up into the air by themselves without effort, and this imagery began to take effect. She had once suffered from a total lack of function in the deltoid muscles of her upper arms, but now these muscles were becoming noticeably thicker and stronger, until at last she could raise her arms. When she was able to do this and had practiced it for two months, we gave her some "weights" to lift: first a grapefruit, then a cantaloupe. By that time, Rivka could work on herself steadily for hours at a time, without needing constant prodding from us. Left alone, she would continue to exercise, and when we came back she would still be at it.

After receiving her new braces, Rivka's development speeded up greatly. When she first got them, we started to take her for walks before dinner and then invite her to eat with us. At first, she could only take about fifteen steps at a time, and I had to carry her down the few steps leading from our apartment to the street. But before long, she could go down the steps by herself, and after a while she was able to walk a whole block — several hundred yards — on her own. I used to tell her not to eat French fries, which she loved — especially not from a deli near our house, where the same oil was used for several batches. But one day when she had walked the half-mile to that deli, where she almost collapsed from the effort, I gave in and bought her a big bag of French fries. She ate them with a pleasure that showed she knew she deserved a treat.

In the beginning, Rivka always needed me near her when she walked, to help maintain her balance and prevent her from falling. She also needed to feel my reassurance and emotional support. Later, she was able to walk alone around the block. Her walking was slow and laborious, but inside she was soaring.

Rivka also began to awaken as a person. She had formerly been indifferent to herself, feeling useless and unwanted. Now she began to feel that she really mattered. She had been almost completely immobile before, able to take only a few steps with braces or on her knees. Now she could get out into the world on her own two feet.

About three months after receiving her braces — and almost exactly six months after my argument with her orthopedist — Rivka made a dramatic leap in her improvement. She could walk half a mile in twenty minutes, whereas before it had taken her an hour and a half. Her walking had strengthened her knee muscles and reactivated her lower back muscles, which had been so numb and contracted that they'd felt like dead flesh. It became easier for us to rotate and stretch her legs and, as a result, Rivka's knees straightened until at last they became completely straight. Rivka began to wear her braces for four or five hours a day, while before she had never been able to tolerate them for more than half an hour.

On top of that, Rivka's formerly paralyzed arms were now fully mobile and growing stronger. We gradually increased the amount of weight she could lift, until it was up to twenty pounds. After six months of wearing her braces, she could walk a whole mile. Once she accomplished this, she worked to increase her speed until she could walk a mile in little more than half an hour — close to normal walking speed.

One of Rivka's greatest triumphs was also one of mine. One day, she arrived late for her session. She was accompanied by one of her sisters, who announced, "We're late because we took the bus today!" Giving Rivka a look of admiration and pride, she added, "You know, this is the first time Rivka has ever taken the bus. She climbed the stairs all by herself." I held back my tears, but my eyes were wet. I carried Rivka up the stairs to keep her from having to make any further effort, took off her braces, and massaged her feet and legs, which were tight from the exertion. I was exhilarated at the thought of Rivka's new independence; she was like a timid little caged bird that had finally been set free.

I thought about the orthopedist's plan to break Rivka's leg. He had never for a minute believed that she could regain function in her legs, never hoped that she would develop her wasted muscles, never imagined that she could do more than take a couple of steps with her braces. Seeing Rivka come to life made the whole world come alive for me and for all of us. Vered said, "You should have made that bet after all. You would have won."

But with or without the wager, it was clear that everybody had won; not only Rivka, not only the three of us, but the world itself had won something in that there was one less crippled child. For it is my deep belief that the suffering of each afflicted person affects the whole world, and that the state of the whole world is reflected in the life of each individual.

PART 2

SELF-HEALING THERAPY

CHAPTER 8

EYE PROBLEMS

During the time when my practice at the Vegetarian Society was flourishing, a woman who successfully improved her eyes with my guidance asked if I would meet her son, Dr. Zimmerman. He was the head ophthalmologist at a hospital where another colleague of mine worked. I was hesitant to see a man whose ideas about treating the eyes were bound to be opposed to my own, but his mother assured me that he was an open-minded person. I later learned that she had coaxed him into meeting me in the same way.

The morning before I met Dr. Zimmerman, I spent a long time doing my eye exercises. Thus relaxed and confident about my work, I let his mother take me to his office. Dr. Zimmerman turned out to be a pleasant young man with a broad, beautiful smile. He listened with great interest to my story and my theories. When he looked at my eyes, he said that he would have done a better job with the surgery, and that my lenses looked like glass that had been dropped and stepped on. Then he tested my vision and simply could not believe how much I was able to see.

Dr. Zimmerman and I disagreed about many things. He couldn't believe that glasses were harmful. I explained to him Dr. Bates's idea that glasses weaken the eyes by preventing them from working for themselves. I also told him that glasses focus more light on the macula (the center of the retina that provides detailed vision) than it could comfortably accept. The concept of eye exercises was new to Dr. Zimmerman, but it made intuitive sense to him. However, he could not accept the idea that the shape of the eye could actually change.

After our conversation, which was courteous and stimulating for both of us, Dr. Zimmerman expressed no great interest in pursuing my methods himself, so we parted as if this conversation were complete and we wouldn't see each other again. His mother, undaunted, decided that if her son wouldn't pursue this with me, she would find another doctor who would. She then talked one of her son's colleagues into trying my work.

Dr. Shem had eye problems himself, and he met me at Mrs. Zimmerman's home. "You can't do anything unconventional at the hospital," she had told me. I taught him relaxation exercises and sunning, and by the end of the session he was so relaxed that he fell asleep. Exercising his eyes was totally new to him.

After the session, Dr. Shem practiced his eye exercises faithfully and experienced some improvement in his vision. This delighted him, not only because of the improvement, but because he felt so bold and adventurous. He continued to exercise for several months, and improved his vision considerably.

I met one other ophthalmologist at Mrs. Zimmerman's home, who told me flatly that eye exercises had no value at all. He said that it was impossible to objectively measure any vision improvements as a result of eye exercises. I found this amusing, since the "objective" findings of ophthalmologic testing vary from day to day and even hour to hour if the tests are repeated. Because they see patients for only a few minutes, eye doctors overlook the constant changes in visual acuity that every individual experiences; they base their knowledge only on what they find in those few minutes. Just about everyone seems to see worse when he or she is tired, overworked, or distressed. Why this isn't generally understood among ophthalmologists is a mystery to me.

Dr. Bates's Approach

WHILE I'M GRATEFUL for the developments in ophthalmology that have helped many, I am concerned that there is no science of preventive ophthalmology. I am sure that Dr. Bates's clear, straightforward theories will somday be endorsed by conventional eye doctors, and not just by the people who improve their vision by natural means. I look forward to the day when ophthalmologists refer their patients to instructors who will teach them prevention and better usage of their eyes.

The Bates method is very effective, and it is based on sound and workable ideas. Bates had an approach that genuinely helped people to cure their eye problems — and not just common eye problems, but some serious degenerative eye diseases. He didn't consider his findings to be in opposition to the spirit of his profession, but rather a means of widening the horizons of ophthalmology. However, no profession has ever welcomed sweeping changes in its practices. Bates was not only discredited, but he lost his license to practice ophthalmology. Though his ideas were rejected by conventional ophthalmology, he continued to help thousands of people to overcome their eye problems. Pioneers in any field are often persecuted and forced to fight for what they consider worthwhile and true.

Bates always emphasized that his method was not a fixed set of techniques, but should be adjusted subtly to meet each individual's needs. While describing his exercises, he also said that if a patient was not helped by the exercises in his book, that person should try to develop new exercises by experimenting, as Bates himself had done. Bates understood that there was no one technique that would help everyone. Relaxation is the only consistently effective factor.

Bates also explained that eye problems could result from worry and stress, as well as from an unhealthy environment. Environmental factors that may be harmful to vision include poor light, noise, air pollution, and a lack of distant horizons that give the eyes a chance to "stretch."

Boredom is another factor. When we are bored, we tend to stop focusing and let our eyes "glaze over." This habit, which may lead to myopia and astigmatism, often begins in childhood. The typical classroom is a very unhealthy atmosphere for the eyes. Children spend six hours a day in an enclosed, artificially lit space, trying to pay attention to lessons that are frequently boring or frustrating. They begin to stare vacantly or let their eyes wander aimlessly, and that blurs the vision and may cause errors of refraction, such as nearsightedness or astigmatism. It is no wonder that so many children who enter school with perfectly healthy eyes need glasses by the time they are nine years old.

Aunt Esther Comes Around

AT THE AGE OF EIGHTY, my aunt Esther was in a car accident and broke her leg. She was bedridden for three months while the leg was healing; at the end of that time, a neurologist told her that she had Parkinson's disease. He recommended that she have physical therapy to prevent her joints from stiffening and degenerating.

Aunt Esther telephoned me and asked if I would be her therapist. My schedule at that time was full, so I gave up my morning exercises at the beach to work on her. I enjoyed those sessions at the beach immensely, and I knew that Aunt Esther would be a difficult patient, but I really couldn't turn her down. As it turned out, she was completely uncooperative. She wouldn't work on herself outside of our sessions. She accepted the treatments as her due and wasn't interested in how she might enhance them.

When I first came to see aunt Esther, she wasn't able to get out of bed. After a month of loosening her joints and reducing her tremors through relaxation exercises and meditation, we began to walk together; I showed her how to walk properly. One time, we walked to a lovely wooded area near her house that had a small stream. As we sat down on a bench, aunt Esther asked me, "How is it you know so much?" It was as if she knew nothing about the years I had been working on myself and others. Only after she felt the effects of my work herself did it occur to her that my endeavors might have some validity. It impressed her that this treatment had gotten her out of bed in just one month.

I told aunt Esther about Miriam, Isaac, Shlomo, and the many other people I had worked with. This seemed to make sense to her, but she said, "You still should get a degree in physical therapy." When she had suggested this several years earlier, it was her way of denigrating my work. But this time she said it respectfully, to encourage my obtaining credentials so that this work might be accepted more widely.

Aunt Esther's illness brought us closer. We both enjoyed the time we spent together. She felt less need to control me, and she increasingly indicated that I was doing the right thing. She was particularly impressed when she learned that half a million people had listened to my interview on the radio. At the end of her treatment, aunt Esther presented me with a wonderful gift: a plane ticket to America.

I knew that my best chance of earning official credentials was in

America. I also realized that going to America would put me in contact with a much greater number of people. I had begun to feel that my practice had gone as far as it could in Israel. Our center was nationally known, thanks to the radio show and extensive publicity by word of mouth. Despite long hours of work, Danny, Vered, and I couldn't see all the people who wanted to see us. It occurred to me that becoming better known and accredited would allow me to train or influence the work of other practitioners, making our therapy available to more people. I wanted to eventually set up a hospital where our method could be used.

Going to San Francisco

MY SISTER, BELLA, had been living in San Francisco for some time, and she suggested that I join her there while pursuing a graduate degree in physical therapy. But two conventional schools of physical therapy in Israel had already rejected me: One refused to accept me because of my vision, and I'd made the mistake of telling the admissions committee at the other about my work. I feared that, even in the United States, my method would be opposed. So I compromised and decided to go to San Francisco for two years to complete my undergraduate education, then return to Israel.

Bella met me at the airport and took me to her home. I could barely believe it was really happening. I felt as if I embodied the thousands of miles I had just traveled from Israel to America. As I went to sleep on Bella's couch, it seemed as though I were still up in the air.

It took me about a week to realize that San Francisco really was a totally different place than Israel. The most striking difference was that I had no patients. I had the strongest urge to work; being unable to work was the worst fate I could imagine. It was incredibly quiet. At home in Israel, the phone rang every five minutes, and I would meet friends everywhere. I felt as though I was wasting time when there was so much to be done.

I'd had so much support from physicians in Israel that I decided to contact doctors in California to see if one might help me get started working here. I had absolutely no success. Some were polite but couldn't imagine how to help me, and most dismissed me without a word.

Meanwhile, Danny and Vered continued their work with clients at our center in Tel Aviv. I missed them a lot, so we arranged to stay in touch. Because phone calls were expensive at the time, they would send me their recorded letters on cassette tapes, and I'd call them back to talk about their clients.

Finally, after six months, I received a letter from Israel with the phone number of a teacher of the Alexander Method (a type of bodywork) in California. We arranged to meet, and he told me that he would do his best to refer patients to me. He also introduced me to an optometrist he knew named Dr. Raymond Gottlieb.

Dr. Gottlieb was the first person in the United States who seemed to understand and appreciate what I had to say. He had an excellent practice, but he felt dissatisfied with it. "I myself practiced Bates's exercises," he said. "I had a slight myopia, and I improved it within a year and a half. Now my vision is normal or better. But I feel that the real experience of it evaded me, even though I worked hard and improved my vision." I knew what he meant. "Maybe you worked too hard at the exercises instead of just experiencing them," I suggested.

I gave Dr. Gottlieb a few treatments. His abdomen was very tight, and I helped him release the tension by contracting and then relaxing every muscle there, and by massaging and stretching each of his limbs. I stretched his arm while he visualized it reaching across the room, the street, the ocean; this relaxed his shoulders and chest. Afterward, he stood more solidly on the ground and his face was more relaxed.

With his initial approval of my work confirmed, I began to go to Dr. Gottlieb's office one day a week to work with a few patients. The people I saw turned out to be quite interested in my work and the exercises, but most of them were not at all diligent about practicing between sessions. They were open to new ideas, but they really did nothing substantial with them.

I began to notice that people with low self-confidence tended to take a stance of general defensiveness, while people who were confident could put their full effort behind what they were doing. The latter were much better able to improve their vision and their health. As I began to better understand the new people I was working with, my work and results improved.

Dr. Gottlieb's friendship and support were tremendously important to me. He opened the doors for me by introducing me to the holistic healing community in the San Francisco Bay Area. During this time, I decided to drop my plans to study physical therapy and focus on my own work. I realized that the classes I had been taking helped me better explain the concepts behind my method.

A few months after I began seeing patients in his office, Dr. Gottlieb and I opened a therapy center together in San Francisco. He encouraged me to teach vision-improvement classes there. Until then, I had only worked with individuals, and I wasn't sure my work would be effective with groups of people. I soon found out that, in a small class that met for three or four hours, I could establish an atmosphere of closeness and give each student individual attention. Everyone who stayed with the course improved his or her vision, but some people found ingenious ways to avoid plunging into something unfamiliar. My method demanded that the students change their whole way of seeing, and some people responded by calling the work difficult or time-consuming and leaving the course in the middle. Over the years, fewer and fewer students left my classes early, but I think I was a little too brash and direct during those first years in the United States.

Still, I found that I could teach students how to develop kinesthetic awareness along with conveying the basic principles of my work. The classes were a success. Dozens of students completed them and improved their vision.

I am grateful to Dr. Gottlieb for helping me get started in the United States. After several more months of working together, he and I had learned what we were able to learn from one another, and we went our separate ways. At that point, I opened my own Center for Self-Healing in San Francisco. I was twenty-three years old. It was several more years before I founded the School for Self-Healing, dedicated to teaching the Self-Healing Method.

As time went on, working with individual patients became my main activity again; I didn't need to lecture or explain so much. My touch offered patients relief and strength, and they usually didn't concern themselves with the theory behind it. Still, the experience of teaching was valuable for me; I learned how to talk about my work in a way that inspired people to care for their eyes and their bodies.

Luelia: Healing Body and Eyes Together

LUELIA WAS my first major success in America. She was a seventy-year-old woman who complained about headaches, redness and pain in her eyes, and a stiff neck and back. She told me that she'd suffered from crossed eyes and double vision since birth. She'd been going to a chiropractor, sometimes twice a day, as well as a homeopath and an ophthalmologist. In addition to her chronic problems, she had periodic eye infections. Luelia was hypersensitive to light, and she worried incessantly about her health. Whenever she came to see me, she always had a list of a dozen health problems. Despite her complaints and her loneliness, she had a lot of courage and many interests. She was the editor of a small publishing company that specialized in religious books. She was a very religious person, and in this she found her strength and comfort. She believed that her coming to see me was divinely ordained.

Although Luelia had adjusted to seeing double, her eyes were in constant pain from tension that couldn't be relieved by drugs. She had even worked with Bates teachers, but her work had been unsuccessful. She finally gave up on both conventional and holistic methods and decided "to put her problems in God's hands."

Luelia found me by a circuitous route. She'd been visiting a museum outside Los Angeles when she met a tourist from San Francisco who asked her if there was something wrong with her eyes. When Luelia told the woman her story, she said, "The best Bates teacher in the country lives in San Francisco. He helped me overcome my arthritis." Then she gave Luelia my address, which was three blocks from where Luelia lived. She was sure that God had provided an answer.

Luelia called me from Los Angeles the following day, and the next Sunday, instead of going to church, she came to see me. A small, frail woman with snow-white hair, Luelia had been taught by a so-called Bates Method teacher thirty years earlier to suppress her stronger eye and use only the weaker one. The teacher's intention had been to strengthen the weak eye, but forcing it to function for both eyes had put an intolerable strain on it; in the process, Luelia had weakened her good eye by underusing it. When one suffers from double vision, each eye sees a separate image and doesn't fuse the two into one. Telling Luelia to suppress one eye was completely wrong; she needed to learn to use both.

Luelia also told me that another Bates Method teacher had insisted that she try to see a tiny dot on a page, and yelled at her when she couldn't see it, but gave her no further instruction. Many people who teach the Bates Method have confused and distorted ideas about his work. When Dr. Bates said that it was necessary to see even the smallest details with clarity, he didn't mean that we should strain and force ourselves to do so; he meant that we should be able to learn to use our eyes in such a way that this would become possible. For Luelia, it was especially wrong to strain her eyes to see.

Luelia also suffered from insomnia; she never slept more than two hours at a time. She told me that no one could massage her without making her scream in pain. Her body was very fragile, with many ruptured blood vessels and weak muscles. I massaged her so gently that, at first, it was hard for her to feel anything; she wasn't even aware that she was numb.

On top of her serious physical problems, Luelia was nearly paralyzed with anxiety; she could never relax. She wasn't able to palm her eyes because leaning her elbows on the table made her fear that she would injure her shoulders. I didn't insist that she palm, but instead I told her to sit in a very dark room, close her eyes, and imagine that she saw blackness.

It was important that I not impose a discipline, but gradually introduce Luelia to this work and let her proceed at her own pace. She needed to be able to decide what was right or wrong for her, even when I disagreed.

I suggested to Luelia that she allow her double vision to return, then alternate using each eye. If it was necessary to use one eye more than the other, she should use the stronger one. Soon she was able to read and type for more than an hour without becoming tired. Within a month of working this way, the redness in her eyes cleared up and the irises became crystal clear. Whenever she was tired, she sat in a dark room and tried to see black. This relaxed her and relieved any pain. Her tolerance to light increased, and she squinted less. Soon, Luelia wasn't afraid of palming.

After a few months, Luelia's initial purpose in coming to me had already been accomplished: She no longer had incessant pain, and she could type for hours. However, I wanted her to change not only her symptoms, but her fundamental problem as well: her overriding tension, caused by fear. Her tension was so bad that, several times when she was riding in a car that passed over a small bump, she dislocated a vertebra and pinched a nerve. Her body was so tense that anything could harm her, and she was terrified of this. I needed to help her strengthen and relax her body so that she would be less susceptible to fear.

As time passed, Luelia began to participate more in her healing, both mentally and physically. Her tension slowly lessened, and her tissues began to regain sensation. It is essential for everyone to exercise so that the tension that accumulates in the muscles can be released. This was especially true for Luelia.

I taught Luelia simple, gentle movements for her muscles, and after a while she could practice forty minutes each day. She told me that this was the first time in her life that she'd ever done any exercises consistently. "Exercises usually just tire me out. But yours are different; they really help me." Whenever she began to get a headache, she would gently rotate her head from side to side. She learned to massage herself, and she learned to release her lower-back tension with gentle leg exercises and deep, relaxed breathing. For the first time, Luelia felt that she was in charge of her own health. In fact, she developed such confidence that she began to tell me what to do during our sessions.

Luelia became considerably less susceptible to pinched nerves or a stiff neck, and her eyes improved remarkably. We dedicated one session every two weeks to her eyes. Sitting at the large window of my office, Luelia would look across the street at a shop sign. At first, she saw the letters double, but overlapping. I asked her to close her eyes and imagine that the distance between her and the sign decreased. She was to block out all other details and focus her attention on the sign. Then I asked her to open one eye, look at the sign, close it, and then do the same thing with the other eye. As she looked at the sign, she shifted her focus from point to point; after a while, she became able to distinguish the center of her visual field from its periphery. Although the image still wasn't clear, paying attention to her peripheral vision relaxed her eyes, and she could distinguish a letter or two and see the spaces between the letters. When Luelia opened both of her eyes together, she saw everything distinctly double. This showed that she was beginning to correct the habit of suppressing one eye, and it was a relief for both eyes.

Then I had Luelia open one eye, look at the sign, then close the eye and imagine the sign as having very black letters on a very white background. She did this, first alternating eyes, then finally with both eyes together. Soon she was able to see the whole sign clearly with each eye individually. Then I told her to close both eyes and imagine that she saw the sign, first with one eye and then with the other eye, and then to imagine that she saw the sign from an angle with each eye separately. Finally, I asked her to imagine fusing these two pictures into one. When Luelia opened her eyes, she could see — for a few moments —

one clear, perfectly legible image of the sign. She was utterly amazed! From that time on, her vision improvement accelerated.

As Luelia's eyes relaxed more, they ceased to be crossed. This indicated that her cross-eyed condition had resulted from tension. Sunning and palming, mental visualization exercises, and learning to look at things without effort combined to correct her vision. The idea that seeing required effort had been ingrained in her. To break this habit of straining while looking, I taught Luelia blinking exercises. Straining to see inhibits a person from blinking enough, and not blinking leads to further strain. If you try to look at a point without blinking, even for a minute, you will see how much effort this requires. Blinking rests the eyes and is essential for good vision.

I also asked Luelia to take a pen and move her eyes up and down along it as she drew a line with it. If she had looked at the line, she would have made an effort to see that the line was drawn straight. Seeing the line only peripherally, she could draw it without tension and consequently drew it straighter. She repeated this exercise daily; it helped her learn to relax while seeing with her central vision because she had become familiar with relaxing while using peripheral vision.

Luelia eventually stopped using her glasses altogether. She was permitted to drive without glasses, and she stopped getting eye infections. Her double vision from birth permanently disappeared at age seventy-two. You cannot help the body without helping the eyes, and vice versa. Luelia is a superb example of this.

Donald: Regaining Vision after a Stroke

DONALD SUFFERED from double vision as a result of a stroke to his midbrain. For years, he had eaten all the unhealthy foods, although he knew better. He was a compassionate, effective, open-minded psychologist who had suffered a lot of turmoil in his own life. At the age of fifty, after the stroke, his vision was no longer functional. Fortunately, he came to see me only four days after his stroke, before his brain learned to accept the damaged vision as natural.

When Donald sat down facing me, he saw a double image of me. He quickly relaxed, because he felt comfortable with me. I also found myself relaxing in his presence, for I realized that he would be friendly and cooperative. I was therefore immediately able to find the right

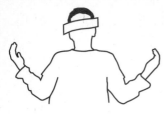

exercise for him: I taped a long piece of construction paper horizontally to the bridge of his nose to block his central vision, then I asked him to wave his hands where he could see them in his peripheral vision. For the first time in four days, he didn't see double and didn't feel that his vision was compromised. The effect was temporary, but it gave him a sense that he could do more. I also taught him palming and sunning.

Donald's uncoordinated, uncooperative eyes caused him unbearable stress. To help him, I taught him an exercise using red and green glasses. One of his eyes would look through a red plastic filter while the other looked through a green one; this separated the visual tasks of the two eyes. Then I showed him a red circle drawn on white paper; this could be seen through the green filter, but it was invisible through the red filter. I then handed him a flashlight with a red light. Because red light can penetrate a red filter but not a green one, he saw the circle with one eye and the light with the other. Now the real

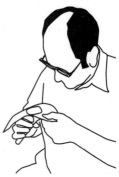

exercise began: I asked him to hold the red flashlight under the paper with the red circle, and to try to trace the circle with the red light. People whose eyes work in coordination can do that without difficulty. Donald was off by 12 inches; his eyes just could not work together.

Using bodywork, I helped relax Donald's face and increase the circulation to his head. We patched his strong right eye. His right eye had been dominant all his life, so his eyes hadn't worked well in coordination with each other even before the stroke. In my opinion, the stroke exacerbated a dysfunction that had been present in the first place. In Donald's case, as in many others, in times of crisis areas of weakness suffer the most.

Donald was sometimes impatient with the exercises and tried to save time by combining several. Since the stroke motivated him to lose weight and get in better shape, he started exercising on an exercise machine: a ski simulator. While exercising, he wore a decorated crown that his wife made for him, with colorful ribbons hanging from its sides. The ribbons would wiggle and move as he exercised, stimulating his peripheral vision. This stimulation sent a message to his brain that both of his eyes should be working at the same time. This eventually also helped his central vision.

With his right eye patched, Donald practiced throwing and catching a ball again and again to activate his lazy left eye. Stimulating the left eye led to its active participation in seeing. All of a sudden, Donald was able to see a single image in the center of his visual field.

At that stage, Donald found that he was developing single vision in the distance, but was still seeing double at close range. We then began to work outdoors. Standing at the top of a hill, we divided the vista into three parts: The far portion was three blocks away and beyond; the middle portion was a block away; and the near portion was about a yard away from him. Looking into the far range, he could see a single image. He would then gradually look at objects in the middle distance until he saw double. He then looked far away, then again closer toward the middle distance. His double vision in the middle distance decreased within about ten minutes, and disappeared within twenty. He then repeated the exercise, shifting his focus between the middle distance and the nearby area. He would rest by palming for a moment every once in a while. After practicing this during a few sessions, Donald was able to see a single image even from nearby.

Donald went away for a couple of months. When he returned, he reported that he was seeing partially single and partially double, and that he was learning to live with it. I heard despair in his voice. I asked him why he said that, and he said, "I talked with a woman who has double vision from a stroke. She told me that, yes, some neurologists think that double vision can be self-corrected, but the truth is that it really never corrects itself, so you just learn to live with it. So I decided that I'm going to learn to live with it. After all, I'm a psychologist." "That is exactly what you don't want to do," I replied. "You don't want to learn to live with it; you want to know that you can overcome it."

We continued to work, finding that bodywork and movement helped Donald see single images because of the improved circulation to his eyes. We worked on strengthening his external eye muscles to make it easier for him to look forward with both eyes. We started to work with an exercise using a string and beads: We had several beads, each a different color, threaded on a long

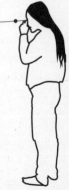

string. We'd tie one end of the string to a post. He would then stretch the string between himself and the post, hold the other end of the string at the bridge of his nose, and focus on one bead at a time.

When the eyes work in coordination with each other, the brain combines the images created in the central vision of both eyes, while the images created in the periphery remain different from each other. If your eyes are well coordinated, you can demonstrate this to yourself by holding one of your fingers vertically in front of your face, about a foot away from your eyes. Close one eye at a time, and you'll see your finger at different angles, appearing to be in different places. Open both eyes, and you'll see one three-dimensional finger; your brain has combined the images from both eyes into one. The brain doesn't do that in the periphery. This is obvious in the areas where the visual fields of both eyes don't overlap: If you hold both hands up at the sides of your head, about 3 feet apart from each other, your left eye will be the only one informing your brain about your left hand, and vice versa.

What is not so obvious is that, even in the area right in front of you that both of your eyes can see, the brain only combines the images of the object you are directly looking at. Everything else, even if it is close by, is regarded as "periphery" and is not combined into one image. To demonstrate this to yourself, hold your two index fingers vertically in front of your face, one of them 8 inches away from you, the other about 10 inches behind it. When you look at the farther finger, you'll see two separate images of the finger that is close to you, and vice versa. Only the images of the finger you are looking at are combined by the brain into one image. The other finger is regarded as peripheral vision, and the images of both eyes are not combined.

Similarly, if you were to look at beads on a string, and if you have the capability to focus both eyes on one bead, you would see the other beads as double. The beads you are not focusing on directly are seen by both eyes as being in the periphery. Donald found this string-and-beads exercise very challenging because his brain could not unite the images of the bead he was trying to focus on. He managed, with practice, to see a double image of the beads he was not focusing on, and he learned to move his focus from bead to bead, but for a while he couldn't see any one bead as a single image. Eventually, he was able to see the bead he focused on as one single object, while the peripheral beads were double. He started to realize that, when he was able to distinguish between the periphery (everything he wasn't looking at) and the center of his vision (the specific bead he chose to look at), he could fuse his vision in the center. The more he could see a difference between what his two eyes were seeing in the periphery, the better the fusion in the center.

Donald ended up overcoming his double vision, except for one little corner on the left side of his visual field. He didn't complete his therapy, but he improved by more than 98 percent.

Daphne: The Power of Commitment

DAPHNE CALLED ME and said that she was suffering from double vision after a bad fall. I recommended that she come in right away, and she did. Not everyone responds so quickly; Daphne was very motivated and ready to work immediately.

Daphne told me what had happened: She had gone to pick up her daughter at a friend's house, and she'd walked down the stairs to their basement carrying her three-year-old son in her arms. She didn't realize that the stairs were under construction at the time. She'd only taken a couple of steps when she tripped and found herself falling forward. She could only think of holding her son tightly; she couldn't hold him and protect herself with her hands at the same time, so she hit the concrete at the bottom of the stairs with the right side of her face. She screamed for help. Her friends came immediately, told her that her little boy seemed fine, and somehow helped her up the stairs to the living room. She sat there with a splitting headache, afraid to open her eyes, until the emergency medical technicians arrived. When they asked her to open her eyes, she saw double.

Daphne had fractured her right orbital bone. After a week, when the swelling had subsided, she'd undergone surgery to repair the fracture. Her eye doctor had told her that the double vision might go away — but then again, it might not.

When Daphne came to see me, she devoted herself to working on her vision without hesitation or reservation. She was both fortunate and wise to start her exercise program within weeks after her injury. As in Donald's case, her brain hadn't yet accepted the double vision as a way of life; she hadn't adjusted to it as she would have if she'd waited longer to begin therapy. This was the best window of opportunity for a cure.

Daphne saw double when she looked up, right, or left, but not when she looked down, and — much like Donald — not when looking ahead into the distance. During her first session with me, I asked her to look into the distance for forty minutes to relax her eyes. In most cases, the eyes are more relaxed when looking far away, and this was especially true of Daphne because it gave her relief from double vision. It is distressing to suffer the blur of double vision on top of feeling the lack of control that accompanies it.

Daphne's next step was to alternate between looking into the distance, where her eyes worked well together, and looking a little closer — halfway between herself and the horizon, where her vision was double. She'd look back and forth, hundreds of times, between the horizon and halfway there. She worked on herself for hours every day doing this exercise, then for another hour or two during her daily sessions.

Gradually, Daphne overcame the double vision while looking forward; she could look forward at any distance with both eyes and see a single image. When she managed to not see double looking forward, we worked on looking to the left. She would see double there, then shift her gaze forward to where her vision was now clear, then again to the left. It took many hours, but she was persistent and had the same results: She could now look to the left without seeing double. Then she started to alternate between looking forward and down and left and right, gradually increasing the turn to the right. After one very intensive week of working with me, the only area where Daphne still had double vision was looking up.

I suspected that, in addition to the trauma of breaking the orbital bone, Daphne had had a concussion. I believed that her double vision had to do with her brain's perception, not just her eye misalignment. We had to wake up the nerve cells whose job was to coordinate the work of both eyes — those cells that were not damaged.

Six months after Daphne worked with me, I called her and learned that her double vision was almost totally gone, even in the upward direction.

Daphne is a true self-healer. Although she had an injury, shock, and a family to raise, she cleared her head and worked to overcome symptoms that could otherwise have remained a hurdle for the rest of her life. She had a positive attitude and a strong will, and she was able to achieve excellent results.

Nancy: From Blindness to Vision

ONE OF THE BEST EXAMPLES of the body's power to heal was Nancy, an eighteen-year-old Canadian Indian. Her parents accompanied her on her visits to me. Her mother, who had heard about my work, was happy to bring her daughter to see me. Her father — a strong, tall, pleasant man and a leader in his community — was apprehensive and suspicious about bringing Nancy to work with me. They told me that Nancy had suffered from a thyroid problem, and that one of many results was an undeveloped optic nerve. Nancy said that her left eye was legally blind; she could see 20/200, or 20 percent of normal, with it, and could read from no farther than 2 inches. Her right eye was completely blind, except for color and light perception.

I sat and chatted with Nancy and her mother for a while, then Nancy looked at the eye chart. Her vision tested at 20/100, which is 50 percent of normal vision, rather than the 20 percent of normal vision that she'd previously tested at. "We went to all the top specialists in Canada," said her mother, "How come she didn't see better on their charts?" "She is so relaxed now," I replied, "that her vision is at its best. At the ophthalmologists' offices, she was probably tense, so her vision wasn't measured at its best."

Our first exercise had to do with stimulating Nancy's weaker eye. We patched her stronger, left eye with thick black paper, all the way from her nose to her temples, and from her forehead to her cheekbone. I didn't use a normal eye patch because I wanted no light whatsoever to enter her left eye. I also asked Nancy to cover her patched eye with both hands. In a totally dark room, I turned on a blinking red lightbulb. Normally, people with vision as poor as Nancy's would be able to tell that there was some light in the room and that it blinked, but they might not be able to tell where the light was located. In about a minute, Nancy saw exactly where the light came from. A minute later, she could see the shape of the lightbulb. A minute after that, she saw my general features. Two minutes after that, she was able to describe my face. All three of us — Nancy, her mother, and I — were completely taken by surprise. It was a powerful experience for us all, especially for Nancy, who couldn't yet comprehend what had happened to her.

Apparently, in all the clinical tests, Nancy's strong eye had been covered for just a moment before her weak eye was tested. In my experience, with cases like Nancy's, it takes about three minutes of covering the strong eye completely before the weak eye starts to see.

We then went outside for our next exercise, with Nancy's strong eye still covered. I asked her to bounce on the large trampoline while catching and throwing large colorful balls. She felt weird, out of place, and unbalanced; she had never, ever used her right eye. Now she was catching and throwing balls using that eye alone.

For a whole week, we spent time during each daily session walking up and down the street with Nancy's strong eye patched, looking at large signs and other objects with the weak eye. At the end of the week, we measured the vision in her weak eye as 20/400 from afar, while her stronger eye improved to 20/60 (70 percent of normal). Her vision was much closer to normal than it had ever been.

Nancy's father watched in amazement as she and I sat in an almost-dark room, with her strong eye patched, rolling a ball back and forth between us. He was so impressed that he encouraged her to return the following year. Nancy worked on her vision at home between her visits to me. During her second visit, we completed the work on her eyes by developing some fusion — eye teaming that creates depth perception.

Basic Bates and Beyond

IF YOUR VISION is less than perfect, there's a pretty good chance that you're straining to see. Street signs, freeway signs, business signs, printed menus, books, newspapers, and homework all assume that your vision is excellent.

If you learn to use your vision without straining, you'll find that it can improve. It doesn't matter what vision problem you are dealing with; even if your vision will always remain limited, it can be better than it is now. Maybe the structure of your eyes won't change, but then again maybe it will change over time. Even if the changes in your vision won't be measurable on an eye chart, the improvements can be substantial in terms of the eye-brain-body connection. Vision is largely achieved by the brain, and only partially by the eyes.

As I mentioned earlier, Dr. William Horatio Bates was an opthalmologist in New York at the beginning of the twentieth century. He observed that people's vision is not fixed, but varies constantly with the time of day, the stage of a person's life, and emotional changes. Vision can become worse, but it can also improve. That understanding set Dr. Bates apart from the medical profession, which believed that vision is a fixed phenomenon, predetermined by the structure of the eye.

Dr. Bates identified a few principles and developed several exercises, three of which are explained below. The first principle was to not strain; straining, in his opinion, leads to poor vision.

Palming

This is the main exercise Dr. Bates used to relax the visual system. Tibetan yogis used this exercise as a form of meditation; they knew it improved their vision.

Rub your hands together to warm them, close your eyes, and put your palms over your eyes. Remember the color of total blackness. Dr. Bates even used the memory of blackness as a tool to overcome pain.

Swaying

This exercise promotes relaxation and opens up the peripheral vision.

While looking at a fixed point, swing your body from side to side. You'll have the illusion that the object you're looking at is moving in the opposite direction.

The Long Swing

Again, move your body from side to side in a half-circle, but this time let your eyes follow wherever your nose is pointing. You'll have the feeling that the whole world is going in the opposite direction.

When you get this sense of movement, your brain is stimulated to explore, to move the eyes from point to point. This exercise, therefore, reestablishes the *saccadic* movement of the eyes — the quick, almost imperceptible exploration of details that the eyes tend to do when they see well. The long swing also stimulates peripheral vision, relaxes the central vision, and thereby allows the eyes to move quickly and easily from one small detail to another. When saccadic movement is done well — at about seventy little automatic movements per second — there is no blur.

Dr. Bates also explored "shifting" — keeping the gaze moving all the time. You can learn to shift your gaze between smaller and smaller objects, such as between the lines on an eye chart. Shifting also develops the saccadic movement that I just described; it breaks the habit of staring, which is common among nearsighted people.

Dr. Bates also recognized the importance of good lighting. It's important to explore what lighting conditions are most comfortable for your own eyes.

Many eye exercises and techniques have been developed since the time of Dr. Bates. "Sunning" is one such exercise. Sunning helps relax the eyes, stimulate the retina, and exercise the muscles of the iris so that the pupil can shrink as needed. I recommend practicing sunning early in the morning or late in the afternoon.

Sunning

Close your eyes, face the sun, and move your face from side to side very slowly, so that your chin points toward one shoulder and then the other. Alternate between sunning for a few minutes and palming for a few minutes, and you may find that the darkness becomes very deep when you palm.

Massaging one's face, especially around the eyes, is another later addition to vision-improvement programs. Using hand-eye coordination exercises, such as blocking the strong eye and playing ball using the weaker eye, are also tools for more specifically addressing one's needs.

Many practitioners have added concepts, techniques, and exercises to the array of vision-improvement methods available. Much has also been learned since Dr. Bates's time about the connection between stress and vision loss.

You can also use the exercises that I've described for stimulating the periphery and enhancing binocular vision. When you block your central vision with a piece of paper, then wave your hands at the sides of your face such that each eye sees one hand, you encourage both eyes to work at the same time, without competition.

How to Improve Your Vision

YOUR VISION CAN IMPROVE. I say this with confidence, even if your eye doctor tells you otherwise. It doesn't matter whether or not your vision can be corrected by glasses, whether your vision loss has been minor or you're almost blind, or whether the source of your problem is genetic, environmental, injury, or poor use of the eyes; you can take the next step toward using your eyes more efficiently.

First, acknowledge how much vision you do have. As my colleague Aileen Whiteford, from Scotland, says: "You never have poor vision, you never have bad vision; you always have good vision. All vision is good, and improving it is a matter of working on it." She would even have you look around the room blindfolded, just to appreciate how much vision you do have when you remove the blindfold. You may be more aware of what you don't have than of what you have, but simply acknowledging your capacity is powerful — and much more truthful to your soul.

How can you care for your eyes? Be aware of the strain that you impose on your eyes, and give them a chance to rest from it. Using the eyes for near vision is hard on them — and so many of us do that almost all day long. Give your eyes the opportunity to look into the distance, without glasses or contact lenses on — permitting the blur if it's blurry — just to give the ciliary muscles a chance to rest and to allow your lenses to be flat for a while. If you're using a computer, which is harder on the eyes than reading a printed page, remember to blink, remember to breathe, look into the distance as often as you can, and pay attention to your peripheral vision; don't limit yourself to the confines of the monitor in front of you.

Electric lighting also strains your eyes. You may not have many choices about the lighting in your workplace, but if you do, try to use full-spectrum light or at least explore what lighting conditions are most comfortable for your eyes. And, while you may like the ambience of dim light around your house, your eyes will appreciate strong light much better.

Glasses are no cure for poor vision, and they offer no relief for weak eyes. Some people think of glasses as crutches; I think of them as harmful. Think about your last visit to the optometrist: You probably sat in a poorly lit office, looked at a poorly lit eye chart, and worried about whether your vision would turn out to be worse than the previous time you had it tested. The lighting conditions and your anxiety provided an excellent setting for you to be at your worst. Then you were fitted with a pair of glasses that were just right for you — when you're at your worst. But you're not always seeing that poorly; you use those glasses when the lighting is good, when your eyes are relaxed, when your mind is at ease — all of these being times when the glasses are just too strong. How do you manage this overcorrection? That's easy to guess: You blur your vision to adapt to the glasses.

Recent research has shown that wearing glasses for nearsightedness, farsightedness, or astigmatism may exacerbate the eye problem that the glasses were prescribed for in the first place. But that isn't all. Using glasses to correct nearsightedness has been shown to limit the use of peripheral vision; that alone is enough to increase one's nearsighted-ness. But glasses do even more; they distort the speed at which objects move in one's visual field. It's no surprise that nearsighted people tend to stare, concentrate on details rather than the whole picture, and fail to respond to movement in the periphery of their vision.[1]

Are contact lenses any better than glasses? They don't limit eye movement as glasses do, and they don't limit the use of peripheral vision as much as glasses do, but they deprive the cornea of oxygen, they teach the eyes to tolerate foreign objects, and they put the cornea at greater risk of laceration.

I recommend that people who are working on improving their vision replace their contact lenses with glasses, primarily because they are more likely to remove them for a little while now and then. If your vision was corrected with glasses to 20/20 or better, get yourself a pair of glasses that corrects you to 20/40 instead; you need to be able to read, write, and drive, and that correction is likely to be enough. Keep your stronger glasses for driving under difficult conditions or other situations in which a reduced-rate prescription may cause you strain. Not every optometrist is open to prescribing glasses with a reduced prescription, but some will. You may want to look for a behavioral optometrist in your area (contact the School for Self-Healing for referrals to behavioral optometrists and self-healing practitioners in your area). If your vision wasn't correctable to 20/20, keep the glasses you have until you can see better with them before changing to a lower prescription. After you've practiced the Bates eye exercises and conscious relaxation of your eyes for a while, you'll find that your vision, using the reduced prescription, improves. When you see 20/20 with your reduced-prescription glasses, get a new pair again, with an even lower prescription.

---

[1]Anna Bambridge, "An Investigation of Myopic Visual Function and the Effect of Holistic Vision Therapy," Masters of Philosophy thesis, 2001, Vision Sciences Department, Glasgow Caledonian University, Scotland; and Anna Bambridge, "Approaching Myopia Holistically: A Case Study and Theoretical Exploration," *Journal of Alternative and Complementary Medicine*, vol. 8, no. 3, 2002, pp. 371–77.

It is a challenge to remove your glasses and not strain to see as well as you did with them. Even in a safe setting, such as sitting on a chair and looking into the distance, you may find yourself making an effort to see all the details you know you are missing. Take a deep breath and make a conscious decision that none of those details are worth the strain. Allow yourself to have blurry vision, forgive yourself for having blurry vision, and be patient. It may help if you think of your field of vision as your own personal artwork: Today it may look like a watercolor when you're looking into the distance. The first step in the process of learning to see better is learning to look at the world without straining. If you can do this much, you will find your vision improving. It may be a long process, but it's worth the wait.

I'm often asked for my opinion of sunglasses. Many people who spend a lot of time indoors under artificial light, or just poor light, find outdoor sunlight intolerable. If you find yourself squinting in the sunlight, it's because your iris muscles have become too weak to constrict your pupils. Don't reach for your sunglasses; they're like crutches that promote dependency. Your pupils need to learn to constrict, because during the day tightly constricted pupils allow for much better vision than pupils that are wide open.

How do you teach your pupils to constrict? By practicing the sunning exercise. You'll be amazed at how fast you'll overcome your dependency on sunglasses. You may want to keep them for extreme conditions, such as skiing or driving facing the sun, or for use after trauma, dilation, or taking certain medications — but not for regular use.

But there's more than that. The retina needs sunlight to function well. There are pigments in the eye that absorb the light that enters through the pupil. I fear that sunglasses tamper with the work of those pigments. I am concerned that sunglasses will be found to contribute to degenerative ailments of the eye, such as macular degeneration.

People also often ask my opinion of surgery, such as LASIK, to correct vision by changing the shape of the cornea. Of course, I'd much rather see people address their eyestrain — the root cause of their nearsightedness. In addition, people who are nearsighted may be prone to problems such as retinal detachment; surgery of the cornea doesn't reduce that risk, and time will tell if it actually increases the risk. But there's more to it than that. I urge you to learn about the possible failures of cornea surgery; I see them all the time. I meet people who saw well after the surgery — for a year — and then their vision deteriorated again. I meet people who had to give up driving at night, people whose eyes have become so sensitive and dry that they suffer from frequent pain and infections, and people whose vision can no longer be corrected (even with glasses or contacts) to the acuity that was available to them before surgery.

For those who insist on going through with cornea surgery, I have some important advice: By all means, don't let your surgeon convince you to correct one eye for near vision and one for far vision. When the eyes can never work together, the eyestrain is tremendous.

Current ophthalmological theory is that eyes cannot improve, even with exercise. Do your eye exercises, teach your family and friends, and show your opthalmologist something that he or she doesn't know. Eyes do change, they change constantly, and they can always change for the better.

CHAPTER 9

BACK PROBLEMS

Over the past thirty years, I have seen more than 2,000 people with back problems of many kinds. Most have shown remarkable improvement after learning correct movement. In my experience, all back problems can be greatly alleviated or completely cured by understanding how the condition developed, then using proper exercises, breathing, and massage to relearn how to use the spine correctly.

I agree with most doctors and health-care practitioners, who believe that back problems are caused by injuries. However, I am convinced that excess weight, tension, or stiffness can make a person more injury-prone. If your body is tense at the time of injury, the injury may be more severe — and the recovery slower — than if your body was relaxed. Most people use the whole back for every motion, as if the back is a single, inflexible entity. The back is comprised of individual vertebrae and small, separate muscle groups. It is natural and healthy to use the back flexibly, not rigidly. If you use the muscles of the back to do the work of the limbs and other parts of the body, you create unnecessary tension in the back and unnecessary rigidity in the limbs. The brain gets the message that the back needs to work when it actually doesn't, and that the limbs do not need to work when they actually do.

When I first examine a spine patient, I look at how the patient walks, particularly whether the walk is balanced. Proper gait and balance require proper use of the body's exact physical center, which is located in the area around the navel. If a person always operates from that gravitational center, the person's posture and spine will be straight and the movements of the body will be perfectly balanced. Problems such as imbalance, gait difficulties, and chronic back tension arise when the "center" of movement is shifted from the abdomen to some other part of the body.

To understand this concept, imagine throwing a softball. The force needed for this action comes primarily from the shoulder. The energy, or impetus, for throwing gathers in the shoulder and is expelled all along the arm, into the hand, and into the ball; it is this force that moves the ball. This is how the center works; it is the focal point where the energy needed for an action gathers, and the point from which that energy is directed into the rest of the body. Naturally, using our actual physical center as the center of movement is the easiest, least stressful, and most economical way to move.

However, in many people the center of movement has been shifted — due to incorrect movement patterns — to some other part of the body, such as the chest, neck, or shoulders. When this happens, movement becomes difficult, awkward, and constrained, rather than easy and natural. The energy needed for movement is then drawn from an area that was never designed to meet that kind of demand, and the false center will take the strain whenever movement occurs.

For many people, the "center" of movement is in the back of the head; the muscles and nerves in the back of the head are called upon to direct and provide the impetus and energy for movement for the entire body. This will cause the head to be drawn forward or backward from its normal upright position, tightening the neck and spine and preventing full respiration. Chronic tension in the lower back will result, drawing the back into an exaggerated S-shape — one that is stiff rather than flexible, pliable, and variable with changes in posture.

A slightly exaggerated S-shape has become so common that it is considered normal, but it is in fact the source of most spine ailments. It leads to blockage of circulation, nerve stimulation, pinched nerves, and tense muscles. Spinal curvature of this kind pushes the pelvis forward, cramping the abdominal cavity and interfering with the activity of the internal organs. It limits the expansion of the lungs, inhibiting full respiration.

Similarly, tension can reduce the curvature of the spine. This can be the case with tension in the lower back, the gluteus muscles, or the waist, or it can occur in connection with a ruptured disk in the lower back: The spine straightens in an attempt to protect the injured area.

Operating from One's Center

MIRIAM TAUGHT ME to recognize where a person's center was by observing how they stood. If we don't stand and walk so that all our weight is distributed evenly on every part of our feet, we are automatically off center, and the imbalance will be reflected in all our movements. Many people walk predominantly on their heels, or on the balls of their feet, or on their toes. The part of the foot that receives the most pressure determines where the person's center is. If I walk predominantly on my toes, my center will be in my neck or in the back of my head. If I throw my weight onto the balls of my feet, my center will be in my chest, causing my upper back to curve out sharply. In some cases, this may lead to a hump or a swayback.

The first step in correcting such problems is mental awareness. I always begin by explaining to people which part of their body they've been using as the center. Then I show them where their center should be and instruct them to develop a kinesthetic awareness of that true center. I ask them to visualize their true center and feel its location. Sometimes simply placing their hands over their abdomen and breathing deeply is enough. I ask them to be aware of the feelings of constriction and strain that accompany a misplaced center of gravity, and to replace those feelings with a sense of expansion and lightness. I ask them to relax their head, neck, chest, and especially whatever part of their body has been operating as the substitute center.

The second thing I look for in new patients is how they sit. Spine patients tend to sit with their backs and heads bent forward or curved backward, with their weight more on one buttock than the other.

Third, I notice how patients lie on a firm surface: whether their back is relaxed, or if the small of the back is tensed so that the lower back curves upward. From these observations, I can tell how a person's back problems developed.

My Work with Back Problems

WHEN I EXAMINE a new spine patient, I try to locate all the sore spots on the body and massage them until they are no longer painful. Sore spots indicate muscle tension caused by lack of movement. These are likely to be places where emotional tension is stored. Often, I find places that are extremely tight and sore that the patient didn't even know about until I touched them. It is important to show the patient how to breathe freely and deeply into the abdomen so that the back can expand and be in constant movement while breathing. With constant movement in the back, there is little chance that it will become tense and stiff.

Gabi: The Unbearable Weight of Pessimism

MY FIRST BACK PATIENT was a French Israeli named Gabi, whom I met through Shlomo at the beach. Gabi was an intellectual and a philosopher with an extremely pessimistic outlook. He felt that he was often cheated in business. He was also a compulsive womanizer, and had been married and divorced six times.

Gabi was rarely satisfied with anything, and this expressed itself in his posture. He dragged his feet when he walked, placing his weight on his toes and giving the impression that his body was a burden. His center was in the back of his neck, as his back was continually hunched over. He was often tired.

I met with Gabi on and off for two years. Each time I worked on him, the massage relaxed him so that he felt better for a day or two, but he soon reverted to his habitual, heavy way of walking. His brain would issue familiar instructions, and the wrong muscles — those in his lower back — would become unnecessarily involved in his walking. This would cause renewed back pain, and he would begin the cycle again.

Like many people who are not aware of the cause of their difficulties, Gabi continued to use a few overburdened muscles in a forced, strained way, remaining unaware of the burden his body was to him. Massage relaxed him and helped him breathe better, but he never exercised on his own to reinforce this improvement. I respected and liked Gabi, and wished I could have helped him more, but his pessimistic, rigid view of life stood in the way of his total recovery.

David: Releasing Burdens

A MAN NAMED DAVID came to see us after attending one of my lectures. He believed in preventive medicine and was angry at doctors because their drugs and surgery hadn't alleviated his back problems.

David lived in a small port town near Tel Aviv and worked for the telephone company. A tall man, his rounded shoulders and slumped posture portrayed how weak and small he felt. His spine had a pronounced S-shape, and his legs and stomach were tense. His main weakness was in the middle of his back, between the lumbar and thoracic vertebrae. This is often a weak area in people who suffer from low self-esteem. David was inspired by my lecture; he saw in me the triumph of someone who could have remained helpless and weak, but had not. He felt that he, too, could overcome his disability.

We taught David a series of nonstrenuous movements to relax and gently activate each joint and muscle of his back. We taught him how to sit and stand properly. The best exercise for him was a visualization exercise that he would do after preliminary massage and exercising. He would lie on his back on the table with his eyes closed and imagine that his head was very heavy (in fact, attached to the table), that his legs were also very heavy, and that his spine was lying perfectly flat against the table, pulled down by its own weight. After experiencing this heaviness for a while, David would then imagine himself as weightless. This gave him the sensation that he could float away. He would then lie on his side while I massaged his shoulders, and I would ask him to imagine, for a moment, that I was massaging each of his vertebrae. I did this because I wanted him to have a better sense of connection with his back. He could feel the muscles in his back loosening and relaxing as he visualized this. Sometimes imagination is even more effective than massage for relaxing tight muscles. I touched every part of his body: forehead, skull, back of the head, cheeks, neck, and so on. I left my hands on each part for half a minute, telling him, "Be aware of this part of you. How does that feel? Be in touch with it: What sensations is it experiencing?" This helped him get back in touch with the body from which he had become detached.

Then I asked David to be aware of all the emotional pain that was stored in his chest muscles, and to feel the tension he carried in his diaphragm, under his shoulder blades, and in his solar plexus, rib cage, and lower abdomen. I asked him to picture his abdomen as red, then as white, as though redness were pouring into it and flowing out again. I asked him to notice the relationship between his fingers and toes, and to think about how the body connects them. He would then imagine blood rushing into his legs, all the way to his toes, then up his legs again into his stomach, rib cage, shoulders, and arms.

After doing that exercise, David always felt as if a heavy burden had been lifted. By becoming more aware of his tension, he learned how he might also relax. He encountered all the obstacles in his life, and he became able to direct his newly released energy toward creating a healthier life. He became astute at noticing tension as it arose, and he served as his own therapist in relieving it. After only six months, David gained enough confidence and experience that he didn't need to see us anymore.

Helping Mr. Shadmi Tie His Shoes

I MET MR. SHADMI, a retired general, on a summer day, during my afternoon break. Most people in Israel take a break from work between 2:00 and 4:00 P.M., when the heat becomes almost intolerable for some. Danny had just finished making lunch for the three of us. Our lunches always began with a huge slice of watermelon; I bought watermelon daily from a man who sold them from a horse-drawn wagon. On those hot days, I could have eaten whole watermelons by myself.

But just as I was about to join Danny and Vered for lunch, someone came through the door. He was a tall, gray-haired, older man, who greeted me politely, saying, "Hello, I'm Mr. Shadmi, are you Meir Schneider? I've just been talking with Noam, the Alexander teacher [the Alexander Method is a type of bodywork described on page 113]. We were discussing some eye surgery I'm supposed to have, and he suggested that I talk to you before going through with it." "What eye surgery are you supposed to have?" I asked him. "It's an operation to correct my left eye. Do you see how it turns inward?" I came closer and looked at his eye; it indeed turned sharply inward, as though it were trying to look at his nose. He couldn't turn it to look straight ahead. Then I shone a lamp into his eyes and studied them. I noticed red spots on the whites of his eyes, which indicated that they were under a great deal of strain. "Do you have some problem with your sixth cranial nerve?" I asked. "That's right," he replied. "Well, I think we can help you without surgery," I told him. "That would be wonderful," Mr. Shadmi said. "I'd do anything to avoid another operation."

During our first sessions, I taught Mr. Shadmi palming, sunning, shifting, and blinking, the most basic eye exercises. I asked him to tell me about himself, and about what had caused his eye problem. He said, "It happened when I was in the Defense Forces. I was patrolling in a helicopter in the Golan Heights during the Yom Kippur War. I was attacked and shot down, and my body was nearly torn in half. The shock of the fall damaged my sixth cranial nerve. After I was shot down, I took my submachine gun and shot at the Syrian helicopter that had attacked me, and the result was seven broken ribs. The doctors only gave me a 40-percent chance of survival, but I recovered. I had intensive physical therapy, and then someone suggested that I see an Alexander teacher. The Alexander work saved my life. Every night after work, I lie down on the sofa with my knees up, rest my head on a hard pillow, close my eyes, and meditate on extending my back — especially the lower back — and relaxing my muscles. And when I relax, I can just feel my vertebrae settling into place. I feel like I couldn't go on without that."

Mr. Shadmi's work with the Alexander teacher had taught him how to relax, release his muscles, and improve his posture; this made his work with me much more effective. The Alexander Method was one of the first acknowledged bodywork methods created in the West. F. M. Alexander was an Australian actor and singer who lost his ability to perform due to a chronically hoarse voice and stooped back. While trying to overcome these problems, he looked in the mirror one day and realized that he had no kinesthetic sense of his posture; his back felt straight to him when it was actually stooped, and vice versa. As a result, he devised a method of giving mental instruction to his muscles, telling them to become long and soft, improving his posture by directing his neck to lengthen and his spine to flatten. All methods of bodywork aim to do the same things in one way or another: to relax muscles, increase flexibility, and increase awareness of where tension and blockages occur. Many types of bodywork also echo Alexander's assertion that tension in the therapist may be transferred to the patient.

It was obvious that, although he had come to me specifically for eye exercises, Mr. Shadmi needed bodywork just as urgently. He was so stiff that he even found palming difficult, because he couldn't lean forward while sitting. Any forward motion of his back was very difficult for him.

The helicopter accident that had severed Mr. Shadmi's cranial nerve had also shattered his pelvis. Excellent surgery had repaired the pelvis to a great extent, but it had left his back almost immobile. Two vertebrae were fused in his lower back. When he wanted to tie his shoes, he had to lift his feet to where he could reach them with his hands, because he couldn't bend forward. He was often in severe pain.

I massaged Mr. Shadmi's back until it relaxed somewhat, then asked him to lie on his stomach, bend one knee, and rotate his calf. He tried to do this, but was unable to do it smoothly; his leg moved spasmodically in little jerking motions. So I asked him instead to visualize doing the motion; even in his imagination, the leg jerked and twitched. After the visualization, however, he tried the motion again and found that he could do it better. He then repeated the visualization, and was able to visualize doing the motion more smoothly. Visualization exercises demonstrate how much a person's physical and mental states reflect each other.

After this, Mr. Shadmi found that his leg — and, to a lesser degree, his whole body — felt lighter. He was also more flexible, being able to bend his leg farther back so that his calf was closer to his thigh, indicating that his lower back had relaxed somewhat. By the end of our third session, Mr. Shadmi's flexibility had increased so much that he was able to bend over and tie his shoes. Grinning, he said, "Well, it's back to normal life for me. I can actually tie my own shoes. It's a miracle!"

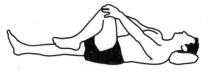

The exercises that had accomplished this miracle were designed to loosen Mr. Shadmi's pelvis. Most of them were done lying on his back. He would bend one knee and cross it over his body to touch the floor on the opposite side, then bring it up again and rest it on the floor on his other side. He would also pull one or both knees up to his chest and move them in a rotating motion with his hands, as shown in the illustration. These exercises greatly reduced the tension in his lower back.

Although Mr. Shadmi did well with the breathing and stretching exercises, he was lax about doing his eye exercises and unwilling to make other changes I suggested, such as in his diet. It was difficult for this busy man to find the hours he needed to work on his eyes intensively. Like most people, he was more willing to give his time to his job or to other people than to himself. I finally stopped teaching him eye exercises, as it was useless without his cooperation. However, I did continue to advise against the eye surgery; it couldn't completely correct his problem anyway, but it would make it more difficult for him if he later decided to work seriously on his eyes.

All things considered, however, Mr. Shadmi's improvement was remarkable. Within eight sessions, he was able to bend over and touch the floor. This was mostly the result of massage. One day he came to me after he had been sitting outdoors on a bench for hours listening to a concert. He felt as stiff as the first day he had come to see me, and he thought it would take several sessions to repair the damage. But after only five minutes of intensive massage, he was able to stand up, bend over, and touch his toes without effort or pain.

Mr. Shadmi told me that he planned to continue exercising for the rest of his life. He appreciated his new flexibility, his deepened breathing, his increased energy, and his greater capacity for deep relaxation. I hoped that someday he would take it all the way, work to improve his eyes as well as his back, and not begrudge himself the hours he needed to work on his body.

Taking Time to Heal Ourselves

MR. SHADMI is typical of modern people; we literally work ourselves to death. In the military, Mr. Shadmi had worked eighteen hours a day. As the head of an electrical company, he now worked thirteen. He would not take time off from work to devote to his health, much less for enjoyment. The pressure was always on.

The irony is that if people take the time to work on themselves, the tensions and pressures of life and work become much easier to deal with. The pressures don't go away, but people who feel relaxed, strong, and capable bring much more to their activities. They can usually accomplish more, and do so more successfully. However, it is difficult to impress this upon people like Mr. Shadmi, who give their lives for their work, their family and friends, and their country — but can't find an hour a day for themselves.

This mentality separates us from the deep inner source of life. This is a great paradox: We sacrifice our lives in order to sustain them; we become enslaved by our ceaseless round of activities. Is this really living? We need to take time to find and develop our inner resources, then bring these resources to our work and our interaction with other people. Everything we do should be part of our development and a step on our journey of self-discovery. Then nothing is done mechanically, and everything is done with new meaning.

I believe that the body is the best place to start; it is a central part of each person's identity. If the body is regarded with reverence and care, this attitude can be extended to the whole self. We need to learn that we are more important than our work, and caring for our bodies can train us in this attitude. Nothing should be allowed to tense our muscles or distort our spines, restrict our breathing or abuse our eyes. And we should learn to value ourselves at a very early age, for it is difficult as adults to change the habits of a lifetime.

Isn't the quality of life as important as life itself?

Naomi's Sunrise

ONE DAY I received a phone call from a man named Yosef, who told me that his wife, Naomi, had just tried to lift both of their twins, and her spine had locked so that she couldn't move. Yosef came to our center to pick me up, and we drove twenty miles to their home. When we arrived, I saw stark fear in Naomi's face; fear and pain were inseparable in her. She told me simply, "I cannot move." She was completely convinced of this. Yet I learned that she was able to get to and from the bathroom by herself. It caused her pain, but because it was a necessity she managed to do it. However, the thought of changing her position from lying on her back to lying on her side, which I asked her to do, seemed impossible to her.

Naomi felt great relief that someone was there to help her. I began to massage her foot. After it relaxed a little, I massaged her leg, then her abdomen, touching her gently and carefully. Her breathing was almost imperceptible at first, but it deepened as I worked. I then massaged her other leg from the foot to the abdomen and, although the pain was still there, she almost forgot that she couldn't move. She was then able to lie on her side as I worked on her pelvis and hips. After an hour, she could lie on her stomach to allow me to work on her back.

Naomi's lower back was so tight that her contracted muscles felt like stone. In her lumbar region, three vertebrae seemed almost fused. I was able to feel the structural effects of her muscular tension. By the end of our three-hour session, Naomi felt looser and her breathing

deepened naturally. She was able to sit up, although with great difficulty. She had some release from her constant pain, but I knew it
wouldn't take much for her to be in pain again.

It was evening when Naomi's husband drove me home. I was
exhausted from the session, and I went right to bed. But my sweet,
soothing sleep was soon interrupted by another call from Yosef. It was
2:00 A.M. He was apologetic, but he told me that Naomi was in severe
pain and asked if I could come see her again. I agreed, but I immediately fell back to sleep. An hour later, I was awakened by Yosef's
knock at my door. He was quite nervous, smoking constantly and driving fast. When we reached their home, I went in to see Naomi; she was
on her back again, her face rigid with fear.

I asked her to concentrate on her scalp. I wanted her to relax through
a slow process of visualization. I asked her to think about the roots
of her hair and the skin that surrounded them, and to allow the skin
to relax. Then I asked her to imagine her breath filling her skull,
and to imagine the skull filling with nourishing oxygen. Naomi became
aware that she was tensing her scalp, and she began to release it. As she
concentrated on her breathing, it deepened dramatically.

I slowly massaged Naomi's toes to relax her foot a little. After
twenty minutes of massage, I could touch her foot firmly. She was
breathing so deeply that she could feel her lower back expand with
each breath. The tension in her foot was connected to the tension
around the compressed vertebrae. In Naomi's foot, I could feel the
pain she felt throughout her body. She gradually became aware of
the source of her pain: the tension in the muscles of her lower spine.
As she breathed deeply, her muscles deeply relaxed; when this happened,
the pain lessened. Naomi's pain was emotional as well as physical; feelings
of helplessness, incapability, loneliness, and inability to communicate
are common to spine-injured patients.

I was now able to move Naomi's legs sideways, apart, and upward
without hurting her. Moving her legs increased the circulation to her
lower back, which was still so tense that I couldn't touch it. When
I asked her to focus awareness on that area, the pain was unbearable.
So I asked her to visualize her hands and feet instead, and to experience their sensations. Focusing awareness in this way tends to
relax the area being focused on, and it increases circulation both
to that area and to the whole body. I massaged Naomi's calves

while she lay on her back, releasing many small points of tension in the muscles. I worked on her knees, one at a time, then her thighs, and then her abdomen.

It was 5:00 in the morning when I started to work on Naomi's abdomen. A little while later, I looked out the window and saw the first red light of morning appearing on the horizon. I told Naomi, "It's dawn already. The sun is just beginning to come up. I wish I could go outside and get a breath of air." She smiled a little. She was feeling some relief from her pain by then, and she said, "Oh, I wish I could, too," and sighed. She couldn't see out the window, which was on the wall behind her bed. Later I said, "The dawn is getting brighter, and some light clouds are moving across the sky." Her breathing deepened as she listened to my description, and she relaxed and was able to roll over onto her side. The first faint red light, which had scarcely been able to penetrate the gray of dawn, steadily brightened until it overcame the darkness and illuminated the whole morning sky. Seeing it through my eyes, Naomi became part of it. The beautiful sunrise renewed us both. Naomi breathed more and more deeply, and her pain diminished. The sky was almost light when her pain finally left her completely. "The moment of dawn is holy," Naomi said to me.

Fearfully, but without pain, Naomi sat up. Then, finding that it didn't hurt, she slowly rose from bed and took three steps without tensing any of her muscles. On the fourth step, her back contracted suddenly; she nearly fell, but I caught her. I showed her how my back muscles would tense if I forced them to participate in the motion of walking, and how they remained loose and relaxed if I didn't. She felt how the different ways of walking influenced the muscles of my back, and she immediately grasped that the same process occurred in her own back. After that, she walked without using or tensing her back muscles. Naomi walked around the bed and stood with me at the window. "It's the most beautiful sunrise I have ever seen, Meir," she said softly. All my hours of work had been worthwhile.

I continued to see Naomi regularly for a year, and at the end of that time she was completely well. Her willingness to see the cause of her problem and to learn a new way of being made this possible.

Getting Bert a Good Night's Sleep

MANY YEARS LATER, in San Francisco, a man named Bert came to see me. He hadn't been able to sleep for two months. He'd been taking steroid medications for asthma, but when he learned that they'd caused him to lose 40 percent of his bone mass, he stopped taking the medications. His asthmatic symptoms returned; he coughed a lot, and he had difficulty exhaling. At one point, Bert coughed so hard that his back went into spasm and he couldn't move. A friend with no experience in bodywork tried to help by stretching Bert's back. After that, Bert was no longer able to lie down and sleep. That's when he came to me.

It took eight careful sessions, bouncing back and forth between improvement and relapse, before Bert was able to sleep for at least three hours a night. He then continued his therapy with one of my colleagues, who was able to help him relieve the back pain altogether.

Building a Healthy Back

WHEN YOUR LIFE gives you a sense of overload, and you feel the burden of your responsibilities, it isn't surprising that the feeling is also physical — right there, in the muscles of your back. By relieving the physical sense of overload, we can relieve the emotional overload that comes with it. Back problems can have many causes, and a sense of overload is only one of them. But all back problems have one thing in common, with very few and unusual exceptions: the tendency of back muscles to contract excessively. Don't immediately assume that you're an exception, even if you have a severe back problem.

Creating and maintaining a healthy back requires continuous work. First we want to be conscious of what muscle relaxation feels like. Then we want to bring that feeling into the subconscious mind. Then we need to search diligently for ways to not contract our back muscles.

What does relaxation of the back feel like? It's a sense of expansion. I recommend visualizing that feeling of expansion often — and everywhere. It's simple: Imagine that your head reaches the sky, your left shoulder reaches to one side of the world, and your right shoulder reaches to the other side of the world. Try to have a sense of that, and keep that sense in everything you do. Write little notes to yourself and post them on your walls, your refrigerator, your computer, wherever you can: "Imagine that the head goes up to the sky, the shoulders expand in opposite directions, and the whole back is expanding."

Back exercises can help you feel this expansion. The following exercise will help you differentiate between areas in your back, rather than using your back as one large block. This is the first step in learning to isolate the muscles used for every movement.

Back Exercise: Differentiation

Lie on your back on the floor; a thin mat is fine. Without using the muscles of your abdomen or chest, press on the floor with different parts of your back. First press with the lower part of the left side of your back, then the middle part of the left side, then the upper part of the left side. Now press on the floor with the lower part of the right side of your back, the middle part of the right side, and the upper part of the right side. This kind of pressure can connect you with areas of your back that you are normally not familiar with. After making this connection, you may find it easier to visualize your back expanding.

Back Exercise: Stretching and Expanding

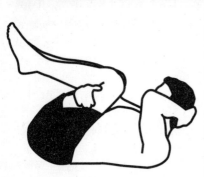

Here's another exercise that helps develop the sense of expansion. Lie on your back, bend your knees, and bring them to your chest. Hug your legs with your arms, and feel your lower back expanding. Now bring your feet back to the floor with your knees still bent, put your hands under your head, and lift up just your head, stretching your neck so that your chin moves towards your chest. Feel the stretch in your neck and middle back. Support your head as you lower it back toward the floor. The third stage of this exercise, shown in the illustration, is to stretch your neck by bringing your head up, this time supported by one hand, and bringing your knees to your chest at the same time, hugging your legs with your other arm.

Back Exercise: Self-Massage for Improved Circulation

Without good circulation, we cannot have a sense of expansion. Self-massage is an excellent way to increase circulation. Here is a pleasant exercise to improve circulation; it can be done while sitting, standing, or even walking: Interlace the fingers of both your hands behind your back and massage your lower back with the backs of your hands by moving them together in circles. Self-massage can also be used on the shoulders: Using your fingertips, knead and tap on your shoulders. As long as it feels good, you're doing it right.

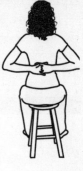

Avoiding Contraction

NOW THAT YOU HAVE a sense of the relaxation your back is seeking, let's explore what it takes to prevent the back from contracting. The most important contribution you can make to the health of your back is to *use the muscles you haven't been using.* The tricky thing is that you may not be familiar with those muscles.

For example, perhaps you find yourself sitting for long periods of time. You may commute to work, travel by plane, or work sitting down for many hours. You may feel discomfort — or perhaps think nothing of it. In both cases, your hip joints, the side muscles of your legs, and your rib cage respond by contracting. What can you do about it? First of all, respond to your tensions. Get up from your seat and stretch every half hour. For example, here's a simple stretch:

Back Exercise: Leg Stretch

Using the back of your chair to steady you, bring one foot up behind you so that you can grasp the ankle and stretch the leg backward and up.

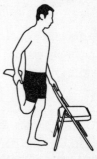

But you can do much more than that. We tend to overuse some of our muscles — usually the large ones — and underuse many smaller ones that are available to us and could help ease the burden. An excellent way to recruit muscles you don't normally use is to walk or run sideways or backward.

Back Exercise: Walk Sideways or Backward

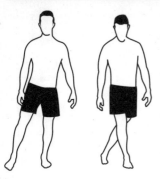

How do you walk or run sideways? You can take a step to your right with your right foot, then bring the left foot next to the right foot. Or you can cross with your right foot in front of your left (have you ever tried folk dancing? Israeli dancing uses this step a lot). Don't forget to do this in the opposite direction, too. If you run or walk like this, even for just 100 to 300 yards a day, you'll open up your hip-joint movement. If you'll be taking an international flight, you owe yourself a quarter mile of this exercise before and after the flight. Do you commute half an hour to work? Save your back and hip joints by running or walking in this fashion no less than 100 yards a day. Try running or walking backward; you'll have to find an open space where you feel safe, and do look back once in a while to see where you're going. You can also modify your walking, just for the sake of changing the muscles you use, by walking forward heel to toe, or backward toe to heel.

When you start to use muscles you haven't used before, the muscles you've been overusing will try to tighten up. In order to prevent them from doing this, maintain awareness of your center. Tap on your abdomen again and again, just below your navel, and try to sense that your center is connecting with the center of the earth. If you can't connect, don't worry about it; just continue with the tapping, and you may feel that your gait is lighter and your head weighs much less.

Separating the Use of the Limbs from the Back

WHAT ELSE CAN YOU DO to soften up your back? Since one of your important goals is to use only the muscles needed for every movement, and to not recruit your back muscles if you don't really need them, then you have to separate the use of your limbs from the use of your back. For example, in the process of getting in and out of a chair, we tend to contract the back. Here's an exercise that will help you understand that you don't really need to do that:

Back Exercise: Standing Up without Using Your Back Muscles

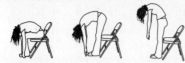

Sit on a chair. Bend forward, bringing your hands to the floor. Still bending forward, get up on your feet as you straighten your legs. Bring the rest of your body up, little by little, lower back first, middle back next, and upper back last, until you are standing straight. Bend forward again, sit down on the chair, and gradually straighten your body. You have now managed to get up from a chair and sit back down without using your back muscles to do so.

Back Exercise: Releasing Tension

Lying on your back, rest your elbows on the floor and move your forearms in circles, as if you are drawing circles with your hands. Keep your wrists loose and let your hands hang from them. Now tap your fingers on the floor for a moment, to have some sensation in your finger-

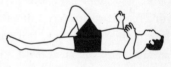

tips. Then imagine, as you resume the rotations, that your fingertips are tied to a puppeteer's strings and are moved around in those circles by the strings. Feel as if there is no need for any muscle at all to get involved in the motion. Now interlace your fingers and move your arms together in large circles to loosen your shoulders. Imagine that your hands are leading the motion. Now lift your head with your hands, trying not to use your neck muscles at all; this will give you the experience of your back lengthening without much tension.

Emotions and Physical Tension

EMOTIONS CAN DICTATE the way you carry your body; we have different postures for aggression, grief, fear, and the like. The opposite is also true: If you arrange yourself in certain postures, you may feel the emotions that go with them. When the back is recruited for movements that could have been done by the limbs alone, it strains, tenses, and holds itself in a posture that reflects a sense of overload. This may be subtle, but it can cause you to carry around a feeling of being overloaded, even if you aren't burdened with a true overload. You may feel a level of emotional stress relating to family, work, or school responsibilities that is greater than your situation really calls for. When contracted muscles in your back give you a sensation of anger, depression, or unresolved feelings, the memories of these emotions may act up — even if there is no current justification for them in your life. If you separate the work of your limbs from your back, you may find these emotions released and gone.

Starting from the Ground Up

WHY IS THE BACK so vulnerable in the first place? Walking in shoes and walking on pavement are to be blamed. Shoes confine the feet, weaken the toes, and immobilize the ankles to some extent. When the ankles become stiff, the knees stiffen. When the knees become stiff, the hip joints stiffen. When those become stiff, so do the back and the neck. You don't have to believe me; try it for yourself. Walk around for a moment with very stiff ankles, just to see what happens when they lack mobility. Can you feel what it does to your knees? Now walk around for a moment with stiff knees; isn't there immediately less movement in your hip joints? Now let's not do any more of that, and concentrate on the opposite. To loosen up your neck, you need to start working on the feet.

Back Exercise: Walking Barefoot

Walk or run on sand or grass, preferably barefoot. Not only are these surfaces softer and less damaging than asphalt or concrete, they are also uneven. They make you step a little differently each time you put your foot down, and that's good for the joints as well as for the leg muscles.

Back Exercise: Working Your Toes

Give your toes the attention they need. Sit on a chair and place your bare foot on the opposite thigh, or sit on the floor and place your foot on the floor in front of you. Using your fingers, move each of your toes in turn, up and down and in a rotating motion, about 100 times a day (not necessarily all in one sitting). Then move the toes against resistance by pressing on them with your fingers and trying to move them in the opposite direction — up, down, right, and left — first keeping all of the toes together, then moving each one on its own. Find out if you rotate your toes independently: Hold onto any four toes, and see if the one you're not holding can rotate.

People who spend much time barefoot usually have stronger, more mobile toes. In my experience, blind people do, too; they often have more space between their toes, which indicates that their toes are more mobile. The reason, I believe, is that blind people walk with more caution, and they depend on the sensation of their feet in order to step safely. We all use our toes all the time, but only partially, and with great tension. It's important to work on relieving the tension and increasing our mobility.

More Ways to Care for Your Back

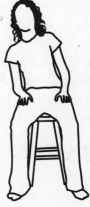

MANY BACK PROBLEMS are a result of neglect. If you have to wear shoes, simply change your shoes two or three times a day. Respond to the strain that sitting imposes on your body by moving your upper body in a rotating motion, like a top centered in your waist. Loosen up your shoulders by interlacing the fingers of both hands above your head and moving your arms in large circles. Find five minutes here, two minutes there, and use them to work on your back: Use a shower massager if you have one; alternate between cold and hot water in your shower to increase circulation; tap gently on your back with a loose fist; breathe deeply and feel your back moving; lie on your back and feel different parts of your back against the floor.

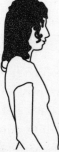

Back Exercise: Tennis-Ball Massage

Here's another thing you can do for yourself. You'll need a couple of tennis balls. Stand with your back leaning against a wall, and keep your feet about a foot away from the wall. Place both tennis balls behind your back, between you and the wall. Make sure the balls are not pressing on your bones — only on the muscles on both sides of your spine. Since you're leaning against the wall, the balls are not likely to fall. Now bend and straighten your knees a little, and feel the balls rolling under your back. By moving your feet farther away from the wall, you can increase the pressure of the balls against your back. Bringing your feet closer to the wall reduces the pressure. By bending and straightening your legs, as well as wiggling from side to side, you can get the tennis balls to massage any area of your back that needs it. You can also place the tennis balls a little higher or lower behind your back, in order to reach to the right spots.

Stay Aware of Your Back

BETWEEN WORKING ON YOURSELF and receiving bodywork, you can relieve tension that you didn't believe you could part from. If you turn the release of tension into a daily reality, your brain will eventually accept this release as your permanent condition.

Whether you have back pain that goes with you everywhere and is present in everything you do, or you're immobilized by pain once in a while, or you just have chronic tightness or discomfort, try to be aware of your back all the time. You can exercise everywhere. You don't have to wait to go to a class, or even to go home and spread yourself on your living-room carpet. Even if you find time to start your day with exercises that get you going, return to working on your back for at least five minutes every couple of hours during the day. If you find a place to lie down and stretch, or even sit and stretch, that's fine. Constant awareness and constant work will help you build a healthy back. Loosen up with every step you make, every breath you take, and every thought you have.

Movement in Many Planes

SINCE MOST OF OUR MOVEMENTS are done in a forward direction (we walk forward, bend forward, lift items in front of us), we need to increase our movement in other planes in order to balance the use of our back muscles. Running sideways, which I mentioned earlier, certainly falls under this category. Here are some other exercises that will help you move in other planes.

Back Exercise: Rolling from Side to Side

One of my favorite exercises is rolling from side to side. Lie on your back and roll from side to side on the floor. Roll to the right until your left hand touches the floor in front of your chest, then push yourself away to start rolling to the left. Then push yourself with your right hand to start the roll to the right. Let your hips and legs also gently push you from side to side. Try to make the movement light and easy, like a child rolling down a grassy hill. Slowly, slowly, the idea of change, of integrating muscles you normally don't use, will sink into your brain. If rolling from side to side makes you dizzy, stop, lie on your back, and gently cover your eyes with your palms for a moment, without putting pressure on your eyes or face. If rolling nauseates you, stop rolling, lie on your back, and massage your abdomen. Abdominal muscles tend to tighten up in just about any movement other than bending forward.

Back Exercise: Shoulder Rotations

If you enjoyed the rolling in the previous exercise, you may want to use rolling as a prelude to these shoulder rotations. Lying on your left side,

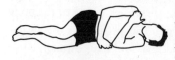

place your right hand on the floor in front of your chest. Move your right shoulder in a rotating motion, about ten times in each direction, visualiz-

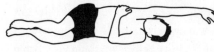

ing the tip of your shoulder leading the motion. Stop the movement and tap on the tip of your shoulder for a moment with the fingertips of either hand. You may find that this makes the visualization easier. Rotate the shoulder again, in both directions. Now tap the fingers of your right hand on the floor a few times, just to have a sensation in your fingertips. Move your whole right arm in large sweeping circles, a few times clockwise and a few times counterclockwise, imagining that the fingertips are leading the motion. Bring your arm down, and repeat tapping on and rotating the shoulder tip. This exercise will encourage your brain to use only the shoulder muscles for the purpose of moving the shoulder and arm, and to let go of your back and abdominal muscles that were recruited unnecessarily. Lie on your back and ask yourself if your right shoulder feels different from your left one. Roll from side to side again ten times, and notice whether your right side is looser than your left side. Now repeat the process with your left shoulder. After completing this exercise, roll from side to side thirty times.

This exercise not only avoids unnecessarily recruiting the muscles of your back and chest, it also utilizes muscles at the side of your body that you normally don't use and helps you integrate these muscles in daily use.

Your Back Exercise Program

IT TAKES DISCIPLINE and self-love to work on the body. But even when we find that space, life still calls for limited use of the body, and the price we pay is the constant creation of tension. When this happens, a mild, sometimes imperceptible depression can creep in and settle into the body. It can take the form of detachment from the body: We may find ourselves going through the motions of our exercises, without really sensing what the body needs or responding to those needs; we may drop our program of exercises altogether. Lack of use of the body leads to even more depression. Be aware of this process, as the awareness itself can help you through it. You may find that, through committing yourself to working on your back and using the gentle exercises your body calls for, you can not only overcome pain, but set different priorities for yourself as well. You may find yourself working toward a sense of well-being and physical comfort before anything else. Being more comfortable in your body will help you resolve other problems. To keep your attention fresh, take it upon yourself to explore a different group of muscles every day; this will keep your work on yourself interesting and make it less routine.

When depression, frustration, grief, and other unresolved emotions are the cause for back pain, allow yourself to actually sense the pain rather than suppress it. Reduce the pain to some extent through movement or massage, but allow yourself to hurt; pay attention to your pain, and let it be your guide. If you numb yourself to the pain, the depression will sink into your tissues. You may be able to work out your pain with a Self-Healing therapist, who will assist you in unveiling it and sensing it. For a while, you may feel your pain to an even greater extent before you can let go of it. If you don't work with your pain in this way, you may find your suppressed pain ruling you and your life. When you slowly relieve the emotional pain, the physical pain will subside, and is unlikely to return.

Even if you work with an excellent therapist, it is your daily practice that will reduce your tendency for back pain. Still, I suggest working with a therapist who is skilled in movement therapy and massage; if at all possible, I recommend working with one who is trained in this Self-Healing Method. First of all, a therapist offers you support. This person can advise you on how to use movement to reduce your tension and stress. A therapist will also offer you love and a warm touch. While psychologists can work with you on matters that distress you, they may not touch you. It has been shown that touch — warm, supportive, and professional — can help relieve depression.

The intimacy of a relationship with a therapist is different from the intimacy of lovers or family. It is an intimacy that energizes and mobilizes you with universal forces. The therapist offers total engagement with your problem and with finding a solution to it, and that makes a big difference. Choose your therapist carefully. Find a person whose own life is a model you appreciate — a therapist who will touch your life in a way that can make an impact. Often, in our lives, we create patterns that are destructive to us both mentally and physically. While common sense tells us to rest, to move, or to sit in a warm bath, our actions will make us work hard, freeze in our posture, and finish that project we took on. The cultural habit of not listening to our bodies is ingrained. Engagement with a good Self-Healing therapist can help you become aware of what you're doing — and make a change.

CHAPTER 10

ARTHRITIS

One-third of all Americans suffer from arthritis. Over the years, I have seen many people with many forms of arthritis improve their mobility and reduce their pain by using my work. It takes gentle movement, massage, and imagery, all practiced with attention and awareness throughout the day.

I use the term "arthritis" to describe a group of ailments characterized by stiff joints and painful movement. The joints of special interest here are the synovial joints, which allow considerable movement between articulating bones — when they're healthy. Where the bones meet, a thin layer of hyaline cartilage covers their surfaces, making the surfaces smooth. The joints are enclosed by a joint capsule, which helps hold the joint together. The joint capsule's structure includes a synovial membrane, which secretes a nourishing lubricating fluid called synovial fluid.

Arthritis involves damage to the cartilage, which can deteriorate and eventually disappear. In arthritic joints, the hyaline cartilage loses its smoothness, becoming rough and pitted so that the bones lose their ability to glide; the bones eventually erode at their edges.

Arthritis begins with pain, swelling, inflammation, and fluid buildup in the joints. In the case of rheumatoid arthritis, an inflammatory disease of the synovium, the immune system malfunctions and attacks one's own tissues (a condition referred to as "autoimmunity").

The synovial fluid and associated connective tissue cells proliferate, forming a cloth-like layer. This causes the joint capsule to thicken, and it destroys the articular cartilage.

Osteoarthritis, the most common type of arthritis, is strongly related to lifestyle. For example, sitting is hard on the hip joints and back. Prolonged sitting can be compensated for by stretching. But in modern culture, most people who live a sedentary lifestyle either find it awkward to stretch or have lost the inclination to do so, whether at work or at home. In my opinion, the stress of incorrect movement of the joints, combined with emotional distress, makes the joints more vulnerable to damage. I also believe that emotional and physical stress contribute to the problem of rheumatoid arthritis as much as they do to osteoarthritis.

Therefore, our work with arthritis emphasizes relearning how to move without stress or undue impact. Using relaxing exercises, we can allow the joints to move to the best of their ability, reducing inflammation and draining off the fluid buildup that causes so much of the pain of arthritis in the early stages. These exercises promote the functioning of the body's innate healing mechanisms. They also lead to more space between the bones, allowing the tissue to repair.

A sensitive touch is particularly important in treating arthritis. A variety of massage techniques and attentive, careful, passive movement of the arthritic joints further stimulate the blood flow and help disperse accumulated fluids. This reduces the swelling and maintains the integrity of the cartilage. The therapist needs to sense exactly how much movement the joints will allow. These gentle movements should be patiently repeated many times while the person receiving treatment breathes deeply. These are the keys to curing arthritis.

Rachel: Relief from Arthritis

DURING MY LAST YEAR in Israel, Dr. Raison of the Vegetarian Society sent an arthritis patient named Rachel to see me. She arrived leaning on a cane and assisted by her husband. Rachel was in her forties, and she appeared miserable and pain-wracked. When she saw me, she said, "You are quite young. But since Dr. Raison recommended you, I suppose it is all right." We joked about this, and she seemed ready to try my treatment.

Rachel had been stricken with arthritis two years earlier, and for a year it affected her whole body. Then the arthritis concentrated itself in one knee, which was swollen to more than twice the size of the other. Most osteoarthritic patients have swollen knees, but Rachel's knee was the worst I had ever encountered.

One of Rachel's doctors had recommended that she have the fluid drained from her knee, but Dr. Raison vehemently opposed this. Rachel became distraught, and begged him to hospitalize her so that she could get the fluid drained. But Raison was adamant: "It would be the worst thing you could do. You could get an infection — or even blood poisoning." "Then give me tranquilizers, please," she pleaded with him. "The pain is so bad I can't even get one hour's sleep at night." "No, you must not take tranquilizers. But there is one thing I can recommend that you try."

He then suggested our therapy, along with a severe diet of organic fruit for breakfast and only sesame seeds, tahini (sesame butter), lettuce, and cucumber the rest of the day. "This diet is unbearable," she confided to me. "The tahini tastes like mud, and the sesame seeds are bitter. Those vegetables are so boring day after day." I was reluctant to criticize a diet suggested by Dr. Raison, especially since it seemed to have brought about some improvement, but the anxiety it produced in Rachel seemed counterproductive.

I began by massaging Rachel's back; I didn't even touch her knee. I showed her how to breathe deeply and told her to visualize a color she liked. After forty-five minutes of deep breathing, visualization, and massage, she was more relaxed and her knee was a bit more mobile. That night she slept for three hours. Then, for several months, Danny took over her treatment; he had the gentlest touch of the three of us. With Danny gently squeezing and tapping the swollen area, Rachel's circulation began to improve and the pain and swelling in her knee lessened. When she first came to us, she had been unable to sleep more than one or two hours each night, and now she was able to sleep six or seven hours. "I am beginning to feel human again," Rachel told Danny.

After Rachel had been in therapy with Danny for four months, I began to treat her again. Breathing exercises were extremely helpful for her; as she breathed in, she visualized the air going into her joints. In just two more months, Rachel didn't need any more treatments. I gave her many exercises to continue doing on her own, including foot rotations, knee movements, and self-massage. After six months of working on her own, her arthritis was imperceptible.

My work with arthritis patients has shown me that arthritis can be improved dramatically just by moving the joints slowly and carefully every day for several hours. If this is done faithfully, the process needn't require more than a year or two. Rachel was willing to devote herself to getting rid of her disease, and she succeeded.

Eileen: Overcoming Physical and Emotional Resistance

TWO OF THE MOST dramatic successes I have had with arthritis came years later, after I established my practice in San Francisco.

One of these patients was a beautiful, dark-haired woman named Eileen. Eileen was a single mother and worked as a legal secretary. In her mid-thirties she had been stricken with both asthma and rheumatoid arthritis. She was taking twelve aspirin a day for her constant, severe pain. A doctor who practiced acupuncture had helped her overcome her asthma, but her arthritis was only getting worse.

Eileen couldn't button her blouse or get herself in and out of the bathtub. Her steps were slow and shuffling, and she had deteriorated to the point where, frustrated by the pain and immobility, she became apathetic about everything — including her four-year-old son. She continued to work, but she only wanted to lie still and be left alone. Her doctor told her that she could expect only further deterioration.

Eileen had two friends who had been my patients, and they both tried to persuade her to see me, but she refused to consider it. Finally, the roshi (head priest) of the Zen Buddhist community where she lived insisted on it, and she came to my office, depressed and pessimistic. Eileen was completely resistant and unwilling to change.

During our first session, I told Eileen that she could be completely cured of arthritis, but she didn't believe me. Anything I could say was contradicted by the swelling and stiffness in her fingers, the constant pain in her toes where the arthritis had started, her stiff, swollen ankles and knees, her immobile pelvis and rigid spine, her congested chest, and the unbearable pain in her neck and shoulders. She was dragging her feet, barely breathing, and hardly moving.

Within a month, Eileen and I reached an impasse. Her refusal to cooperate was frustrating. I began to feel that she was more affected by her disease than she needed to be. It was as if she were cooperating with her arthritis in order to destroy herself. This made me angry. When she dragged herself into my office for our sixth session, her walk was worse than ever. I told her to stand in the middle of the room and lift her leg to rest it on a chair I had placed there. It took her several minutes to do this, and her leg was shaking as if spastic. Then I asked her to bring that foot back to the floor and lift her other leg onto the chair. She had even more difficulty with this. Then I asked her to swing one leg up and over the back of the chair; she did so very slowly, stopping to rest her foot on the seat of the chair on the way down.

When she finished doing this with the other leg, I could barely contain my fury: "If you can swing your leg over a chair that high, why can't you walk without dragging your feet? When I walk, I lift my knees. If I locked my knees and walked as you do, I'd have arthritis, too. No wonder your cartilage is damaged! Stop dragging your feet!"

Eileen was visibly shaken by my tone. "Do you still think you can do something for me?" she asked. "That depends on your willingness to cooperate," I answered. "If you ever walk that way again, I will stop treating you."

After that session, Eileen began to work hard at learning to walk without dragging her feet. She also began to reduce her aspirin intake, and the pain and swelling in her knees decreased. Although it was difficult, she began to lift her knees when she walked, easing the burden of pressure on them, and to coordinate her steps with the movement of her arms. Soon it was obvious that the swelling in her toes, ankles, knees, and hands was decreasing. Although she still felt discouraged, Eileen could see the improvement and understood that she had to learn how to move correctly.

I instructed Eileen to move every joint of her body, including each joint of each finger and toe, in both lateral and rotating motions. At first, this was difficult for her without long sessions of massage, which she had twice a week. When working on her own, however, she would begin by breathing deeply for several minutes and visualizing each joint moving, expanding as she inhaled and shrinking as she exhaled. Thus she worked on both her body and her mental concept of her body. She would count one hundred deep breaths, and with each breath she would "send" the oxygen to a different joint. She worked on the least afflicted joints first — her back, hips, elbows, and hands — rotating and bending, opening and closing her hands.

Eileen's toes and ankles were the most severely afflicted, the first to show signs of damage, and the last joints she would work on. One ankle was so weak that she could actually walk better on it when it was swollen, using the swelling as support. To work on that ankle, she first needed to reduce the swelling, which she did by going to the beach and walking in the shallow water. The cold water not only reduced the swelling, but it increased circulation to that area, making it easier for her to move her ankle and thereby strengthen it.

As Eileen continued to improve, slowly but steadily, I called her attention to many mistakes she was making in movement, from the way she walked to the way she put on and took off her coat. She had been using a few muscles strenuously, and my criticism and teasing helped her realize this.

Eileen was very intelligent. She had a graduate degree in psychology and was studying Zen meditation. At the same time, she felt many emotional conflicts. While she maintained a good relationship with her father, she'd carried a deep anger against him since childhood. She was also angry at the Zen roshi, who had become a father figure for her. She was torn between her wish to submit to a higher authority and her fierce independence and rebelliousness. This conflict left her paralyzed and affected her immune system, causing her white blood cells to attack her cartilage and destroy it. Over the years, I have seen many people suffering from rheumatoid arthritis who also suffered from a severe inner conflict.

Eileen became increasingly annoyed by my criticisms. One day, when I began to tease her, instead of responding verbally as she usually did, she fought back physically. We began wrestling, and I made sure that every joint in her body moved. I lifted her onto the trampoline in our office, and she kicked and punched me as hard as she could. In the process, she was using her hips, knees, shoulders, and neck. Another patient, who witnessed this, said afterward, "I'm not sure that fighting is therapeutic, but it's obvious that Eileen is better afterward!" Eileen, too, appreciated the therapeutic value of our "exercise," but she had also been trying to beat me up. Fighting released some of her anger against me and transformed it into constructive energy. Increasingly, vitality returned to her, and she began to look more attractive and act more concerned about those around her. Even her attitude toward me relaxed, and I felt that it was time for her to begin to really work on herself.

On top of her double load as a working mother, Eileen began to do two hours of exercise every day, moving every joint in her body. She put all her anger into the exercises. Anger became the driving force in her life, and she really came alive. Having begun with extreme apathy, she came to have strong, vital feelings. One day while she was shopping, Eileen noticed that it was no great effort to carry her packages; that awakened in her the realization that she was going to recover. She began to relax for the first time since she had become sick.

The next step for Eileen was using the trampoline to loosen her joints and overcome her fear of movement. A trampoline offers less resistance than solid ground, so bouncing on it is almost effortless. At first, Eileen was afraid of falling, so she sat and bounced on her buttocks, then up onto her feet. Next she kneeled and bounced, first on her knees, and then onto her feet. Each time she did this, she could walk more easily the next day.

Eileen's next step was to stop taking aspirin. She gradually decreased her dosage until she agreed to throw away the aspirin altogether. Soon after this, she became depressed. She wondered why, after all this improvement and increase in energy, she still suffered so much fatigue and pain. By giving up aspirin, she had taken her body out of its state of numbness; the return of feeling made her believe that she was getting worse, even though experiencing her feelings of discomfort was actually an indication that she was getting better. Because she was able to feel for the first time how serious her condition was, she was temporarily overwhelmed by it.

Fortunately, only a few weeks after she stopped taking aspirin, Eileen was invited by her father to join him for a vacation in Acapulco. There, she exercised every day on the beach in the water and the warm sun. She began to feel renewed. Her father, who had not seen her for a year, was delighted with her improvement.

When she returned from Acapulco, Eileen quit her job. She began to swim and exercise in a warm pool, and to work on herself at home for four or more hours a day. She learned to work creatively and with a greater awareness of her body's needs. Exercises in water are designed for freer movement with less gravitational resistance. It is as if the body becomes a part of the water. In addition to the benefits of decreased gravitational resistance, water itself offers a constant, soft resistance that strengthens the muscles with minimal challenge. Furthermore, warm water relaxes and expands the body, elongating the muscles and creating more space between the bones. Exercises that are virtually impossible for an arthritic patient outside of water become easy in water. In warm water, Eileen was able to rotate her feet, open and close her hands, and even walk smoothly.

Finally, two years after we had begun to work together, I told Eileen that she no longer had the rheumatoid factor. She didn't believe me, so I encouraged her to see her physician. When the results of her blood test came back, her doctor confirmed that I was correct. Her white blood cell count, which had been very high, was now completely normal.

While Eileen was still my patient, she often massaged the shoulders, necks, and backs of the other secretaries at her office; she showed such a natural talent that she decided to enroll in my practitioner training course. I had just started offering informal training classes, and I was still surprised that my method could actually be taught. Now only a slight limp remained from Eileen's illness, and her enthusiasm for our work was so great that, in addition to becoming a practitioner herself, she began to address large groups on the subject of self-healing.

However, Eileen still had not resolved her deepest problem: the conflict with her father. She once told me that she had left home in great anger and resentment, determined never to ask her parents for anything. She used all her cash to rent an apartment and get a job; for two weeks, as she waited for her paycheck, she had nothing to eat. One time she was invited out for lunch, and she ate so much that she had to excuse herself and run to the bathroom to vomit. Her escort did not ask her out again.

Because she had never been able to win her father's approval, Eileen never fully accepted herself either, and she always managed to thwart herself when she was on the brink of a great achievement. She would work hard, achieve much, then back away, dissatisfied. After working with me for two years, her body was much better, but the rage at her father had never been resolved; Eileen decided that it was time to sort things out. She stopped seeing patients for a while and devoted herself to her meditation and her Zen community. Her body continued to improve, and her life was happy and full. Within a year, Eileen became married, and she later was appointed secretarial assistant to the roshi.

Then came a fresh disaster: The roshi was accused of wrongdoing, and many in the community turned against him. From being an almost godlike figure, respected by the entire community, he suddenly became the focus of their fears, frustrations, and failings. They had expected so much from him that they could not tolerate his apparent shortcomings.

To Eileen, for whom the roshi had taken a father's place in her affection and respect, this situation created an unbearable conflict. She had a crippling attack, so severe that it took two years for her to recover from it. During that time, I worked on her nearly every day. Even during my advanced training class, in which she was a student, I would massage her ankle as I lectured.

I felt that a cleansing fast would help Eileen, so she and I went off for a six-day retreat in California's Trinity Alps. We stayed in a cabin by a lake and fasted on vegetable juices. I encouraged Eileen to talk for hours about her relationship with her father. On the fifth day, she suddenly burst out, "I just can't see myself getting over this anger! I can't see myself getting strong enough to forgive my father, or roshi. I can't see myself getting well!"

This outburst was very healthy. Eileen had been the victim of her own resentment for years, but she had never before fully experienced it. Now she could experience her rage, not just in her muscles and joints, but also in her conscious mind. I couldn't answer her with words; no words would have helped. But through massage and exercise, Eileen began to cleanse herself emotionally, and at last she could forgive these men.

From that time on, Eileen's health improved rapidly. She resumed her career as a Self-Healing practitioner, and she remains one of the best.

Kristin: Regeneration after Hip Replacement

I MET KRISTIN shortly after she had undergone hip-replacement surgery. Like Eileen, Kristin had rheumatoid arthritis, but hers had progressed so rapidly that at age twenty-five, the cartilage in both hip joints was gone. After an operation in which one worn-out hip joint was replaced with a plastic one, Kristin decided against further surgery. The operation and recovery had been so painful that she was given morphine as a painkiller, and she became addicted to it. Then she was given methadone as a substitute for the morphine, and she became addicted to that instead.

Kristin knew about the Center for Self-Healing before having her hip operation, but had decided in favor of the surgery. Her pain seemed like such a waste to me; I was sure that she could have saved that hip joint.

Kristin was an angelically beautiful, frail young woman. Between pain, hospitalization, surgery, and medication, she had lost thirty pounds from her already slender frame. Her voice was almost a whisper. She leaned on a big, black cane and on the arm of her brother, who had brought her to our office. Kristin couldn't walk without her cane, and her doctor was surprised that she could even walk with it.

In addition to methadone, Kristin was taking anti-inflammatory drugs. She had been given injections of cortisone as well, but these had no effect. Her disease showed in every joint of her body, but especially in her knees, where the swelling was so bad that her kneecaps were hidden beneath the accumulated fluid. She was rigid and stiff and extremely sensitive to cold.

Kristin began our therapy with three sessions a week, each with a different practitioner, and she began to improve almost immediately. Her condition presented some unusual difficulties in treatment. The replacement of her hip joint made it difficult for her to turn over; she had to be moved, and moved very gently. I usually had her lie on her side with her lower leg extended and her upper leg bent at the knee, to stretch out her hip joint. Then I would massage the buttock and outer thigh muscles gently with oil until they were warm. This increased the circulation, not only to her hip joint but all over her body. I instructed her to lie there and breathe, being aware of her lower abdominal muscles as she did so. I showed her how to massage her own hip joint and tap it gently with her fist. I had her lie on her back with knees bent, then move her knees slowly from side to side to activate the inner psoas muscles.

For the first six months, Kristin exercised two hours every day, mostly lying on her back. The purpose of the exercises was to bring circulation into her hip joint area without taxing her body or requiring an effort. I also showed her exercises to do in the bathtub, such as bending and straightening her knees and rotating her ankles. She liked to exercise in the sun, and as the only place she could do this was on the windy roof of the building where she lived, she soon learned to be comfortable with cold breezes and to accept variations in temperature more easily. She even started taking cold showers, which she said made her feel better than anything else. Walking and dressing became easier for her and, encouraged by this, she began to work on herself for three to four hours a day. She felt stronger emotionally and, after a few months, decided to end her dependence on methadone. A hospital-run detoxification program helped her accomplish this.

During a weekend workshop I gave, after two days of working and meditating on her body, Kristin found herself in tears, overwhelmed by emotions she couldn't understand. Those tears must have released something deep inside her, because after that workshop the swelling in her knees decreased considerably, and her kneecaps were visible for the first time in years.

As with Eileen, I took Kristin to exercise in a warm pool. The first time we went, I showed her what it was like to experience movement without resistance to gravity. When she got out of the pool, the sudden return of gravity was so jarring that she could only walk a few steps. At last she was aware of how she put effort and resistance into her every movement. This awareness, more than anything I could say, showed her what she needed to do.

After six months of therapy, Kristin could walk four blocks with her cane. When I first met her, she could barely cross the room! Her doctor was impressed. He said, "Your X-rays show no cartilage in your hip joint. I don't understand how you can walk at all! Whatever it is you are doing, keep it up."

Within a year, Kristin was walking comfortably without her cane for short distances, and within two years, she was able to walk a mile. She joyfully reported each new breakthrough: the day she could sit down on the floor and get up again without help, and the wonderful day when she could get in and out of the bathtub by herself. She stopped using anti-inflammatory drugs and now took only vitamins.

Two years after she began therapy with us, Kristin visited Los Angeles, where she had previously lived. She saw her former doctor, who was a leading rheumatologist. At his urging, new X-rays were taken; when they came back, the results were astonishing. Where earlier X-rays had shown no cartilage and no space between the bones of her hip joint, there was now a clearly visible space. Only seven cases like this were known at that time. Her doctor showed these findings to a group of rheumatologists, none of whom could understand the change. But all agreed that a great improvement had indeed taken place. Those X-rays were an absolute triumph. I had not needed them to confirm Kristin's improvement; I could see it and feel it. But the X-rays served as proof that such an improvement can happen.

I flew to Los Angeles to meet with Kristin's doctor, and he agreed that Self-Healing exercises had been in great part responsible for her improvement. He was not convinced, however, that the space in the hip joint was created by regenerated cartilage; he wasn't ready to believe that cartilage could regenerate at all. Medical opinion stands firmly against this idea, but I have always been convinced that any body tissue can regenerate, given the right conditions. Kristin stands as living proof that even the most severe forms of arthritis can be overcome.

Causes and Relief of Arthritis

THROUGHOUT THE DAY, most people create some stress on their joints. Sitting in one position puts pressure on the pelvis, which may reduce the spaces between the bones in the pelvic area as well as in the hip joint. This can lead to arthritic damage. Our daily life can also be stressful in other ways, at work and at home. In my opinion, when the mind and body have a sense of constant alert, this can trigger the autoimmune response, which in the case of rheumatoid arthritis attacks the joints. Experience tells me that stress reduction is the best prevention against flare-ups of rheumatoid arthritis and the biggest factor in reducing their effects.

The first exercise I recommend uses breath and visualization to bring more circulation to the joints. This exercise is excellent for prevention as well as relief of existing conditions, and I have found it useful even in the most difficult cases.

Arthritis Exercise: Expanding with Your Breath

Lie on your back and support your head with a pillow. You can use another pillow under your knees. Now breathe slowly in and out through your nose. Imagine that your two little toes are expanding as you inhale, and shrinking as you exhale. Visualize the two toes adjacent to the little ones expanding as you inhale, then shrinking as you exhale. Move slowly on to the middle toe, the second toe, and then the big toe, doing the same expansion and shrinking visualization. Now feel as if your breath fills each part of your body, one by one: visualize your feet expanding and shrinking with your breath, then your knees, then your hip joints.

If you have a hard time sensing your hip joints, position your feet hip width apart and roll your legs inward, keeping your heels on the ground, while bringing the toes of both feet toward each other. Then roll them outward, so that the toes of your right foot move away from the toes of your left foot.

You can also give your hip joints a stretch by bending your knees, putting your feet about hip-width apart from each other, and gently moving 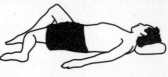 each knee toward the floor between the legs, even if just a little. Feel the stretch in your hip joints, then breathe into the hip joints, first to the right, then to the left, then to both. Visualize your hip joints expanding as you inhale, and shrinking as you exhale.

As you breathe into your abdomen, visualize all your ribs expanding, sense the space between them, then let that space shrink as you breathe out. Now concentrate on your hands, imagining that your fingers and hands expand as you inhale, and shrink as you exhale. Visualize your head doing the same thing. Imagine that you are increasing the space between your skull bones as you inhale, and that the space shrinks as you exhale. When you inhale, visualize more space between your vertebrae; when you exhale, visualize this space lessening. That sense of movement enhances the blood flow.

If you suffer from arthritis and you have a swollen joint, focus on that joint for twenty slow, deep breaths. Inhale slowly and exhale even more slowly, visualizing the joint expanding as you inhale and shrinking as you exhale. In the majority of cases I've worked with, this concentration on a joint reduced the swelling by bringing blood flow to the area. Whenever the mind connects with a joint, the blood flow to that joint is enhanced. If you cannot connect with that joint in your mind, and you find it difficult to visualize, massage it gently for a moment. For example, massage an inflamed finger with the opposite hand, very gently and just for a moment. You can similarly massage your knee, just to have a sense of it, then focus on it for twenty deep breaths, visualizing it expanding and shrinking with your breath.

Restoring Joints

WE TEND TO USE our joints within a limited range of motion, and with much impact. This is an effective formula for wear and tear of the joints. For most people over sixty, the joints of the fingers are often the first to become arthritic. If you look at your hands, you are likely to find that the fingers curve inward; we flex the joints of the fingers, and we need to stretch them in the opposite direction in order to maintain their health. We need to think of the motions we do in daily life, and remember to do the opposite almost every hour.

Here's a simple exercise to move your fingers in the opposite of their normal direction:

Arthritis Exercise: Finger Stretch

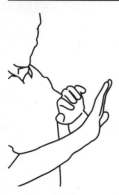

Stretch your hands by extending your fingers, and maintain the stretch for ten deep breaths. Do this several times a day, when you rest or while going about your daily chores. This stretch may bring you a great sense of relief. Also try this: Extend the fingers of one hand and tap on the back of your stretched hand with the fingertips of your other hand. Keep the tapping hand loose at the wrist.

In addition to stretching, here's another exercise that will help your hands:

Arthritis Exercise: Forearm Rotation

Lie on your back on a thin mat or a carpet. Your head can rest on a low pillow or other support, such as a phone book. Rest your elbows on the floor or mat near your body, and rotate your forearms in both directions. At the same time, move your head in a slow, leisurely manner from side to side. Relax your fingers and wrists as you rotate your arms; feel how flimsy they can be.

Arthritis Exercise: Hot Salt Water for Fingers and Toes

If your fingers are swollen and their mobility is reduced, you can use hot salt water to help reduce their swelling. Prepare a large bowl of hot water (100 degrees Fahrenheit), and add to it half a cup of Epsom salt (available at most pharmacies) or salts rich in minerals, such as from the Dead Sea (you may be able to get those at health food stores). If you don't have either, table salt will do. Put your hands in the bowl, open and close your hands ten times, then massage each of your fingers, still under water, allowing two to five minutes for each finger. Now see how your hands open and close. If the water is warm enough and salty enough, you are likely to find that your hands will open and close more easily.

Similarly, you can use salt water for arthritic toes. If you can bend your knee and rest your foot on your opposite thigh, start by massaging the foot and toes in that position. Now put your foot in a large bowl of hot salty water and rotate it (or you can use a bathtub full of water with about three cups of salt in it). If your other foot is arthritic, repeat this with it, too. Rotate your foot in both directions as many as 300 to 400 times; after every 30 or 40 times, stop the movement and visualize rotating your foot. After you are done with the rotations, squeeze your toes together and spread them apart 50 times. At this point, you may find that your toes are less swollen and more mobile, and that you can massage them one by one.

Arthritis Exercise: Shoulder Joints

Here's an exercise for arthritic shoulders: Lie on your back on the floor with your arms straight. The angle 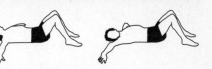 between your arms and your body should be comfortable for you. Now gently rotate your straight arms so that you alternate between touching the floor with your palms and with the backs of your hands.

Don't move your arms any more than is comfortable for you. If your shoulder joints are inflamed, cool them with a refrigerated wet towel to prevent aggravation of the inflammation. To lessen inflammation, you can also imagine that you are breathing into your shoulders, allowing them to expand with your breath; you can also massage them gently.

Arthritis Exercise: Ankle Movements

This exercise is done sitting on a chair. Stretch your legs in front of you, keeping your heels on the floor, and explore the movement in your ankles. Do they move to their full range, or are they limited? Point your toes towards your knees. Does it feel like an effort? If your ankles are stiff, it will be an effort. So go ahead and point your toes toward your knees and notice how your calves, your shins, and perhaps your hamstrings feel. While maintaining this position, take twenty slow, deep breaths in and out through your nose. Now move your feet backward and forward and in a rotating motion in both directions; you may find that your ankles are more flexible. I recommend rotating your feet at the ankles three or four hundred times a day, not necessarily in one sitting. You can rotate them ten, fifteen, or twenty times in both directions just before you start driving, or while you're sitting at the dinner table, in front of your computer, or watching television. If you're not comfortable doing this at work, you may want to teach your coworkers to do this exercise, too, for their own benefit. Take off your shoes, imagine that your feet are expanding as you breathe into them, and rotate your ankles in both directions. These subtle movements are powerful.

Since the feet and ankles are the basis of our standing and walking, these ankle rotations, along with exercises to increase the mobility of the toes, can be the most important exercises for the whole body. The condition of the feet has a great impact on every joint above them, from the knees through the hip joints and back to the neck. The ankle rotations will even make a difference in the mobility of your shoulders and hands.

Arthritis Exercise: Foot Massage

Sit comfortably and, if you can, bring one leg to rest on your opposite thigh. Holding your ankle with one hand and your toes with the other hand, slowly rotate your foot at the ankle. Let your leg muscles relax completely; the foot should move passively, guided by your hand, not using any leg muscles. Stretch your foot as far in each direction as you can comfortably go. Using your fingertips, tap around your ankle and up your shin. Massage your calf with your thumbs. Now rotate your foot by itself, in both directions.

Now rotate your toes. Hold all of them and rotate them together. Now rotate each toe individually: Use your hand to move the toe in circles in both directions, then try to move that toe on its own, while holding the other toes in place. Can you move the toe in circles? Can you wiggle it at all? Most people have an easier time moving the big toe independently, but with practice the other toes can function individually, too. If your ankle or any of your toes can move very little, don't push beyond that. If they cannot move at all, hold on to them anyway and imagine that you are moving them.

Massage the arch of your foot with long strokes of your thumbs, from the toes toward the heel. This can help relax your leg muscles from your toes to your knees. Repeat with your other foot.

The following exercise helps prevent arthritis in the hip joints and knees. Since it promotes circulation, it is also an important exercise if you suffer from arthritis elsewhere, such as in your hands. If your knees are arthritic, you can only use the first part of this exercise.

Arthritis Exercise: Hip Joint Movements

Lie on your back with your head supported by a pillow and straighten and bend first one knee, then the other, thirty times. This will stretch your hamstrings and allow 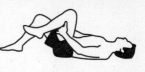 more movement in your knees. Stop the movement. If your knee is arthritic, don't do the next part of the exercise. Instead, just visualize that you are doing it: Bring one leg up with the knee bent, hold your thigh with both hands, as illustrated above, and passively rotate this leg, using your hands, eight times in each direction. Now return to bending and straightening your legs as before.

Arthritis Exercise: Hip Relaxation through Leg Circles

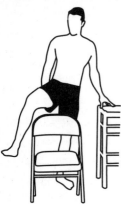

Here is another excellent exercise for preventing arthritis of the hip joint. Select a chair that has a back lower than your hip joint and no armrests. Make sure you also have something to hold on to to maintain your balance during the exercise. Stand behind the chair and tap one of your feet on the floor several times to call your mind's attention to your foot. At the same time, tap with a loose fist on the hip joint of the same leg. Now move your leg in circles around the back of the chair, in both directions. This movement can relax the hip joints and allow good motion in the legs.

Arthritis Exercise: Back Stretches

Stretching the back can prevent it from becoming stiff and arthritic. Sit with your legs folded under your thighs. You might want to put a pillow under your feet, and another one between your calves and thighs. If this position is still difficult, don't do this exercise.

First, stretch the muscles of your chest and abdomen by bending backward. Now slowly bend forward as you stretch your back. Try to isolate the vertebrae, bending forward one vertebra at a time. Return slowly to sitting upright. Resting your hands behind you on the floor, arch your back to bend it away from your left knee. You'll find that this stretching makes it easier to bend forward. Now slowly bend forward toward your left knee. Arch your back away from your right knee. Now slowly bend toward your right knee.

How Joints Function

THE HYALINE CARTILAGE in the joints can remain intact for 150 years — longer than most people expect to live. But these days it's difficult to find a sixty-year-old without joint problems or an eighty-year-old without a serious case of osteoarthritis. This can change, but only if we pay attention to how the body functions.

Muscles hold the joints in place. The space between the joints, which tends to diminish over the years, can be maintained; balanced use of the muscles can keep the joint space large. Our bodies are tired of sitting, tired of walking in the pattern that almost everyone has adapted to, even tired of the way most people practice sports. Many people who engage in sports are just as rigid as those who spend their days in front of computers or slouched on their couches. Try to stay constantly aware of the fact that your body is tired of what you do too much of. Find the best exercises for you — those that take you through motions that are the opposite of what you normally practice. I've mentioned this before, but I'll give you a few more examples. Some of these exercises are similar to those I described in chapter 9, but I give extra instructions for arthritis patients.

Arthritis Exercise: Look Ahead When You Walk

If you tend to look down when you walk, you are walking with a stooped posture, which is very common. Doing this reduces the spaces between the vertebrae in your neck, which can lead to calcification and arthritis. To decrease the chance of harming your neck, all you need to do is develop the habit of looking just a little bit higher than you normally do. A few degrees can make a big difference.

Arthritis Exercise: Walking Well

Because we normally walk forward, exercises aimed at breaking old habits should include walking or running sideways. If, say, you are moving toward your left, let your left leg lead the way and either bring your right foot beside your left foot, or cross your right foot over your left foot. Either way is good exercise. Walking backward is also a good exercise.

When you're walking forward, make sure your foot isn't used as one unit: Bring your heel to the ground and gradually roll your weight to your toes. Pay attention to your knees: As you put your foot down on the ground, the knee of that leg should already be bent. Don't step with a locked knee, as the impact of the step can harm the knee joint. As your body moves farther forward and your weight shifts toward your toes, your knee should bend even more. Straighten only the leg that isn't carrying your weight: the one behind you.

Arthritis Exercise: Sitting Well

If you sit much during the day, explore different sitting postures; joints get tired from being repeatedly put into the same postures. If you sit on a chair or sofa often, try sitting cross-legged, or sit with your legs folded under you (with or without a cushion over your calves). Explore other sitting positions.

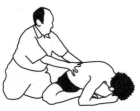

Here is a good sitting stretch (do it only if you can do so without joint pain): Sit on a mat with your left leg bent, your left knee on the mat, and your left foot at your side (not in front of you). Rest your right foot near your left knee and bring your right knee to the mat. In this position, gradually bend toward one knee and then the other. It is even nicer if someone can massage your back as you bend forward.

Arthritis Exercise: Tennis-Ball Back Massage

If you suffer from arthritis of the neck, I suggest using tennis balls for self-massage of the back. Stand with your back against a wall and your feet about a foot in front of the wall, hip width apart. Place two tennis balls between your back and the wall, with one on either side of your spine. Never press on the bones themselves, but on the tight, hardened muscles that run along both sides of the spine. Press yourself against the wall hard enough to keep the balls in place, but not hard enough to cause soreness. The farther your feet are from the wall, the more pressure your body weight puts on the tennis balls. If your knees are not arthritic, you can bend and straighten your knees in this position, allowing the balls to roll up and down along your back. If you find this difficult for your knees, just wiggle from side to side, directing the tennis balls to press where you need pressure. Now remove the tennis balls and place them elsewhere along your back: a little higher or lower. You want to work all the way from your buttocks to your upper back.

Exercising in Warm Water

IF AT ALL POSSIBLE, I recommend that people with arthritis exercise in warm pools (at least 90 degrees). Of course, a warm pool may not be appropriate for everyone; consult with your physician to find out if you have any contraindication, such as multiple sclerosis, a heart condition, or skin problems. Many pools request a release form. If you have no access to a warm pool, exercising in a bathtub or hot tub will have to do.

When you're exercising in warm water, it is important to take a cold shower every fifteen minutes. For example, if you're exercising for an hour, you'll take a cold shower three times during your exercise period, then once when you're done. I am well aware that many people who suffer from arthritis resist the idea of taking a cold shower. But while the warm water relaxes the muscles and creates more space in the joints, it also increases swelling in the joints. Even one minute of cooling can make a difference. As a side benefit, the cold shower is good for your heart.

Following are some of my favorite pool exercises.

Arthritis Exercise: Walking in the Water

Walking in the water is an important form of exercise. It's best if the water is up to your chest, but if it only reaches your hips, it will do. Bend your legs forward and backward, or lift your legs sideways as you walk in the water.

Arthritis Exercise: Bending Arms and Legs in the Water

Stand in water deep enough to reach your shoulders and rest your arms on top of the water. Bending your arms at the elbow, bring your hands toward your shoulders, then straighten your arms again as you open them wide. Repeat these motions for a while. Now lean against the pool wall and continue the arm movements while bending and straightening one leg at a time.

Arthritis Exercise: Climbing the Pool Wall

Face the pool wall and hold on to a bar at the wall, if possible. Climb your feet up the wall — even if just a little bit. Now alternate bending and straightening your knees, one at a time. You may find that this stretches your back, the Achilles tendon in your ankle, and all the way up the back of your legs. You may want to alternate between stretching one leg and the other.

Arthritis Exercise: Leg Swings in the Water

Kick one leg from side to side, swinging it in front of the leg you are standing on. Then change legs. You can support yourself at the pool wall, but you will probably find that you don't need to.

Arthritis Exercise: Passive Arm Movement in Water

Stand in water deep enough to reach your armpits. Rest one arm on the water. Hold the wrist of that arm with your other hand, and move the resting arm passively from side to side. This brings much relief to the passive arm. At the same time, try to kick one of your legs from side to side.

My View of Arthritis Medication

IF YOU THINK that arthritis medication can solve your problems, I disagree. In fact, I don't consider it an option at all. Every year, more people die from medications intended to suppress arthritic symptoms than from all illegal drugs put together. In some cases, taking medication to deal with acute pain may make sense. For example, if you'll die soon and you want to be free from pain, it makes sense to take pain medication. But if your condition is chronic and you take medication, you will need to continually increase the amount you take in order to achieve the same results, and that is just too harmful.

Don't dream of a quick fix. If something sounds too good to be true, it usually is. Drugs may make you feel better today, but then there is tomorrow to deal with: the illness remains, and the body is damaged by the drugs. Read the small print and learn about the side effects of drugs you are considering taking; they are not minor. On top of all that, when the medication makes you not feel the pain, you are more likely to move in a way that can harm your joints. Instead, exercise the pain away, lessen the stiffness through movement, and improve your condition in real terms. Let the pain guide you; take time to let your emotions surface — and then pass. Contemplate, meditate, talk with friends, send yourself good thoughts, and work with your body.

Daily Awareness of Movement

WHEN WE USE THE BODY in an uneven manner, we can expect that, with time, it will wither. Sometimes we have the illusion that the more we demand of our bodies, the healthier they become. Arthritis teaches us that that is not the case. A huge proportion of the population is afflicted with arthritis, but all of it could have been prevented. Many people who suffer from arthritis can overcome it. I wouldn't go as far as to say that everyone can completely overcome all the damage done to their joints, but even very damaged joints can be used better, with more mobility and less pain.

Moving through stiffness can lead to arthritis. Pay attention to what causes stiffness. When we sit too much, or repeat the same motions over and over, or use very few muscles again and again, we can harm our joints. When we pound on our joints by walking and running on hard surfaces or by burdening them with an overweight body, we can damage them. But we should pay attention to other things that lead to stiffness, too: day-to-day stresses; being ill or depressed; eating a poor diet that leads to indigestion, malaise, or fatigue — all these can lead to stiffness, which means limited movement of the joints. We must remember to use more of our muscles, and to move with less strain.

The Role of Stress

STRESS IS AN IMPORTANT FACTOR in the cause of rheumatoid arthritis. You may be familiar with the function of the autonomic nervous system, or the fight-or-flight mechanism, but let's take another look at it in order to make the connection with rheumatoid arthritis.

It is easy to understand the importance of the autonomic, or automatic, nervous system in ancient times. Imagine one of your ancestors suddenly facing a hungry predator many thousands of years ago. What would happen to her body at that scary moment? Her pupils would dilate to let in more light and a better sense of the environment, at the cost of some blurriness in vision. Her heart would beat quickly and strongly, pumping blood to the muscles of her legs and arms. Very little blood would be spent on the internal organs or the skin. Her adrenal glands would secrete norepinephrine, also known as adrenalin. Her body would want to empty her bladder to make running or fighting easier. Assuming that she either defeats the beast by fighting or escapes by running, swimming, or climbing a tree (we did say she was your ancestor, didn't we?), she would then get an opportunity to totally relax from this stress. Her heartbeat and breathing would return to a slower pace, and she would be restored to normal digestion, kidney function, vision, and immune-system function.

Now this is all very nice for jungle situations, but our daily life is normally quite different. While the autonomic nervous system worked well to protect our ancestors from dangers, it also allowed us to achieve real rest from the struggle of survival. While most of us don't deal with wild lions, we may be dealing with other stressors that the body interprets as immediate danger. Financial problems, health problems, legal problems, unresolved personal issues, or terrible national news can trigger the same kind of response in your body as a wild beast would have. But, unlike your agile great-great-great-grandmother, who had the opportunity to resolve her problem both mentally and physically, when you have to live with an unresolved situation and your mind cannot rest from it, your body doesn't get a break from the stress. Even if you resolve your problem, your body may not be able to let go of the stress caused by the situation. Resolving a mental problem mentally is never enough. The problem has to also be resolved physically, or else we continue to carry the tension in our tissues. When the autonomic nervous system is on unnecessary constant alert, it is not working well, and neither is the hormonal system. This is a perfect setting for chronic illness to occur — specifically rheumatoid arthritis, in which the immune system attacks the cartilage of the joints as if they were foreign objects.

It is therefore important to let go of the body's inner stress. On the one hand, you can work on meditating, thinking good thoughts, forgiving even when it's hard, and finding ways to feel better in situations of grief, loss, or other distress. Sometimes you can do this by understanding that the specific upsetting, difficult situations are not your entire life or your entire self; your inner self is much greater than whatever you encounter. But on the other hand, we cannot neglect reducing or eliminating the stress caused in the body. The following are several exercises that will help you do just that.

Arthritis Exercise: Do the Locomotive

This exercise works on the ring muscles that control urinating and defecating. Don't do it if you suffer from a hernia. Before starting the exercise, I suggest that you use the toilet.

Lie on your back with your knees bent. Bring your knees toward your chest, if you can, to relax your legs a bit. Now place your feet on the ground and exhale. Remain without air and alternate between pulling your abdomen inward and pushing it outward several times, keeping your back steady. Now inhale, keep the air in your abdomen, and move the abdomen up and down several times. Exhale, remain without air, and move the abdomen up and down again several times. Relax and breathe slowly and deeply. To relax, inhale and exhale through your nose very slowly three or four times.

Now let's "do the locomotive": Inhale through your nose, close your eyes, and tighten the muscles around your eyes as hard as you can; hold each thumb against the four fingertips of 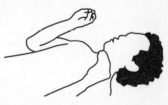 each hand and squeeze them together as tightly as you can; tighten your lips and jaws, and exhale sharply through your mouth with a few forceful "Ch! Ch!" sounds. Inhale again, and repeat the process. This time, after the third "Ch!" sound, don't inhale; tighten the muscles that control your bladder as if keeping yourself from urinating, and hold them for a count of fifteen. Inhale again and repeat the process, this time squeezing your bladder muscles as if you were trying to urinate.

Inhale through your nose. Women can repeat the process while contracting the vaginal muscles, then pushing on the vaginal muscles as if to give birth. Inhale again, exhale, do not inhale, and repeat the process while tightening the anus. Inhale through your nose again, and repeat the process while doing the opposite: pushing as if you were trying to defecate.

If your knees aren't arthritic, continue this exercise standing up (if they are, imagine that you are doing it): Bend forward, then repeat the series of exercises above while remaining bent over; now inhale and exhale through your nose; don't inhale, then puff your cheeks out, let them go, puff them out again, and let go again several times. Now see if you can bend forward farther than you could before.

The idea behind this exercise is that, while we don't let go of stress in normal life, when we mimic the body's physical response to stress we give it the opportunity to really let go of our stress. When the body releases its tension, it truly relaxes and the immune system has an opportunity to function.

To further relax your body, you may now want to repeat the exercise called Expanding with Your Breath (page 142), in which you breathe into each of your joints in turn.

As you can see, if you suffer from arthritis it is possible to increase your mobility. It takes love, care, discipline, and patience. But it's worth it.

CHAPTER 11
MULTIPLE SCLEROSIS

Multiple sclerosis is an autoimmune disease: The immune system attacks and damages the myelin sheath, the fatty tissue that insulates nerves in the central nervous system. As the myelin sheath breaks down, it slows the transmission of messages along the long nerves and makes the nerve impulses weak and ineffective. This disease is considered incurable, although some drugs, in some cases, can slow the deterioration or greatly delay it. Based on results from our own therapy, I know that it is possible for people who suffer from multiple sclerosis to achieve a level of remission that can be considered a cure.

In my opinion, poor use of the body can harm whatever system is vulnerable in a given person's body — the joints, the heart, and so on. People who have a vulnerable central nervous system will find that poor use of their body can cause a flare-up of multiple sclerosis. Although the central nervous system is important in controlling movement — and the myelin is important for fine movement — the body is the environment of the nervous system. Therefore, the body shapes the nervous system and affects its function and health. A typical multiple sclerosis patient has poor posture and a rigid spine. She moves as if her body's center is in her neck, which places great strain in that area. Her back is so tense that the viscera become constricted along with the back muscles. Her whole body is so tight that even her walk is affected. Such extreme tension of muscles and organs leads to neurological dysfunction. Habitual incorrect movement, in my opinion, can damage the myelin. The disappearance of parts of the myelin sheath is simply one of the worst symptoms of misusing the body.

Multiple sclerosis attacks are often the result of a shock or stressor of some kind. These attacks are often followed by remissions, in which some or most of the symptoms greatly decrease. In the case of progressive multiple sclerosis, the attacks that lead to decreased function are not followed by a substantial remission.

Ilana: Overcoming Rigidity

ILANA CAME TO SEE ME at the Vegetarian Society when she was in the early stages of multiple sclerosis. She walked unsteadily with a limp, and her hips appeared to be unbalanced. She experienced numbness in various parts of her body, and she sometimes lost control of her bladder. A public school teacher, Ilana was afraid she might lose her job as a result of her illness.

I started by working on Ilana's right hand and arm, which were partially paralyzed. The muscles she could still use were extremely sore from strained overuse. I taught her a few simple exercises for her arm and worked with her to improve her breathing. Ilana expressed skepticism that any treatment could help her, but as she dressed after her first treatment, she found that she was able to button her blouse without trouble — something she had been unable to do for months. Her arm felt lighter, and she experienced more sensation in it. Since she was doubtful, I suggested that she try just three more treatments to see if they were useful. She agreed, saying, "What have I got to lose?"

I gave Ilana some exercises for her lower back, which was extremely weak and tense. I had her lie on her back with her knees bent, her hands over her chest, and her head on a firm pillow so that her neck could relax. At first, it was difficult for her to keep her knees in this position for more than a few seconds, but after three weeks she could do it for fifteen minutes. I asked her to breathe deeply and count the length of each inhalation and exhalation to help her concentrate on her breathing and keep her mind off her knees. I also asked her to send thoughts of relaxation and expansion into her lower back, imagining it growing wider and longer. Her hips were tight and her ankles stiff, so I asked her to recline in a bathtub full of cool water and bend and straighten her knees alternately, then rotate her feet one by one. The purpose of the second exercise was to strengthen her ankles to increase her stability, and to enhance the connection between her brain and her feet and calves. I also gave her many visualization exercises to help her sense how she used her body: how she moved her arms and legs as though they were extremely heavy, for example, and how her whole body would contract in order to perform one small movement. I wanted to reprogram her nervous system so that it would allow each muscle to do its own work.

Ilana was astonished at the number of changes that occurred during those first four sessions. Her pelvis loosened up. Though it was still difficult for her to walk, she could easily lift her legs to put on her shoes. She went swimming after our third session, and she could hardly believe that she found herself swimming the length of the pool twice; a few weeks earlier, she could barely swim a few yards. Amazed at the changes she experienced so quickly, Ilana consulted her doctor; she confirmed the improvement and encouraged her to continue.

After six weeks, Ilana could lie on her back with her knees bent for half an hour. She even fell asleep in that position once. Her earlier difficulty had come from tensing her knees and ankles. Also, once Ilana's back released its tension, it was free to support itself. Her legs no longer had to work to support her back, nor was their own movement restricted by the tightness of her lower back.

Although the muscles that Ilana was now using had been weak from disuse, they grew stronger as she began using them in a correct and healthy way. Most importantly, she was changing old, ingrained neurological patterns as well as her brain's unconscious belief that her back was weak and her legs were immobile. Her doctor continued to confirm that her knee was getting stronger and that her walk and reflexes were improving. Ilana also made small discoveries on her own; for example, she could sew for the first time in years. All these improvements convinced Ilana that she would be able to return to work in the fall.

Bladder weakness is common among multiple sclerosis patients; the need to urinate can be unbearably urgent and difficult to control. Visualization and sphincter-control exercises proved invaluable in treating this. I instructed Ilana to contract her bladder-control muscles as tightly as possible, imagining that she was holding in urine forcibly. I then told her to tighten the muscles of her upper body as much as possible, including her eyes and mouth, and to forcibly expel her breath through her teeth. Then, alternately, I asked her to repeat the exercise, this time bearing down on her bladder as if she were trying to expel urine but couldn't. (This exercise is described in detail as "Do the Locomotive" in chapter 10.) The exercise helped Ilana achieve control of her bladder, and I have since recommended it to every patient who complains of lack of bladder control.

Vered, who is observant about character and human nature, noticed Ilana's rigidity of mind. Although she was an intelligent, educated woman with many interests, Ilana had inexplicable mental blocks. For example, she was a teacher but she never completely learned Hebrew; she continued to use certain foreign speech patterns that sounded comical in Hebrew. It was as though some parts of her mind weren't in communication with the rest of it. She spoke in a dogmatic way, and she gave the impression of inflexibility in both her mind and body.

Then, as if by magic, as Ilana's body learned to relax and trust, her mind followed suit. She became open to more possibilities, including the possibility of a cure for her illness. Her new attitude seemed to grow naturally out of her new experiences with her body.

I worked with Ilana until I left Israel, and in all that time she did not experience any further degeneration. She never completely lost her limp, but it diminished and her balance improved dramatically. She regained the coordination in her hands, and her mental state continued to improve as she gained trust in herself. It was Ilana who gave me confidence that multiple sclerosis, although an extraordinary challenge, was something we could alleviate.

Sophia: An Unprecedented Cure

SOPHIA GEFEN was referred to us by another patient, named Hannah. The wife of an orthodox rabbi, Sophia was the teacher for the women of the synagogue. Her husband, a kind and unsophisticated man, had done all he could to make her life easier after she was stricken with multiple sclerosis, and he felt much grief about her illness. He drove her to doctors and helped her with errands and household chores. It was obvious that Sophia was deeply loved and respected by everyone who knew her.

The first symptom Sophia had experienced was a lack of sensation in her hands and feet. When she washed dishes, they often slipped out of her hands without her feeling it. Her hands were so lacking in sensation that she didn't even experience numbness. She felt that her hands were immobile and clenched, even when they were open. One day when she arrived home after shopping, she realized that she had the same problem with her feet; she had lost her shoes in the street while walking, and hadn't even noticed it. Tests at the neurology clinic of her hospital were performed by stabbing her hands and feet with sharp objects to the point of bleeding, and she still felt no pain. The doctors confirmed Sophia's worst fears when they told her she had multiple sclerosis.

Sophia was hospitalized and given drugs, but her condition didn't improve and she was released. She and her husband asked her neurologist, "Is there anything in the world we can do?" He replied kindly, "There is nothing medical I know of that will help. Sophia will probably come to see me every six months with another attack and will steadily deteriorate. But don't give up," he added with concern. "You should pray. There is always hope."

From that time on, Sophia was hospitalized every two or three months. Although her attacks gradually decreased in frequency, they increased in severity, and she had no remission or improvement. She was suffering from the chronic, progressive form of multiple sclerosis.

Sophia's balance and coordination almost disappeared, and she was on the verge of paralysis. She could no longer perform any tasks that required hand coordination. When she was able to walk at all, her walking was slow and heavy. At the most, she could walk only the length of her room. Her doctors told her husband that Sophia had no more than eighteen months to live.

A discouraging prognosis handed down by a trusted physician may hasten a patient's death. We have become entirely dependent on doctors for information about our own bodies, our diseases, and our hope for recovery. Physicians should use this awesome power carefully to help encourage their patients, rather than exacerbate their fears. Patients should not treat a physician's prognosis as the only possible outcome.

Sophia's husband and children accompanied her to her first meeting with me, and they were present for our session. Sophia walked in as if her feet were too heavy to lift. She could barely hold herself upright, much less drag herself across the room. Her expression was one of fear, and it seemed to me that this fear was a big part of her difficulty in walking. She seemed to be afraid of each step she took. She would raise one foot barely off the floor, tensing her whole body and face, then she would throw her entire weight onto that foot and drag the other one after it. After a few steps, she needed to collapse or grab something for support. What she feared most was losing her balance. Without realizing it, she was hardly breathing, and the few breaths she took were through her mouth. Her energy seemed almost nonexistent.

I helped Sophia onto the table and asked her to lie on her back. Then, with her knees bent and her feet flat on the table, I started to teach her breathing exercises. As is often the case with severely injured or handicapped patients, she needed to learn breathing first. I asked her to inhale deeply and slowly, then to exhale completely and to wait as long as she could — about twenty seconds — before breathing in again, then to repeat the whole process. She did this about one hundred times.

Sophia soon began to feel her body; she had become completely out of touch with it. The first sensation she experienced was extreme heaviness. She was convinced that the session had helped her, but her husband and children were skeptical, so she decided not to continue treatment. When Hannah heard about this, she visited Sophia repeatedly and finally convinced her to continue treatment with me in earnest. After about two months, Sophia came to my office again. She remembered the exercises I had shown her, and after a couple of weeks of small improvements, she said to me, "Meir, this treatment is a great encouragement." "I hope the effects are not just psychological," I said. "No, I am feeling much better," she replied, "both psychologically and physically, and it gives me hope."

After about a month of working with me, it became obvious to everyone that Sophia's state of mind and body was better. Before this, she had wanted to do nothing. Now she wanted to be involved in as many activities as she could. She was more interested in her condition and was willing to devote herself to her recovery. Even her family began to believe that recovery might be possible.

Sophia's husband was under a great deal of stress because of her condition. Sometimes when he brought her to see me, I would massage his shoulders and neck. One time, I even stood back-to-back with him, took hold of his arms, and bent forward until I was holding him off the floor on my back. Sophia was amazed to see this, as he was much taller and heavier than I was. While supporting him this way, I stretched his arms, neck, shoulders, and back by pulling gently on his arms. This released a lot of his tension, and he was able to sit and relax as he watched our session.

Within two months, Sophia's balance was noticeably better. Although it wasn't consistent or reliable, she tended to fall less. She also had a few hours of relief each day from her constant fatigue. One day, Sophia said, "I feel that something wonderful is about to happen to me." She could foresee a great change. Sometimes when patients talk about the improvement they expect, they are engaging in wishful thinking. But once in a while, a patient speaks about an anticipated improvement with conviction based on deep inner knowledge. When Sophia said that a great change for the better would take place in her life, I sensed that she was right.

From that time on, Sophia's therapy became entirely different. Danny, Vered, and I were no longer working to give Sophia back her health; we just assisted her. The four of us were working together.

Within a month, Sophia began to come to our sessions on her own. She was able to get on and off the bus, and to walk from the bus stop to our office. Although she still limped, her step was becoming noticeably lighter. Walking didn't tire her nearly as much as it had. She felt a renewed sense of enthusiasm, and she began to take walks every day. Her improvements reaffirmed her hope for a cure.

Sophia's coordination was still a big problem. Many simple tasks were difficult for her, and her movements were clumsy and ineffectual. Danny and Vered worked on her until her muscles were relaxed, and I concentrated on giving her exercises. As a result, Sophia's breathing became deeper and more regular, and the increased blood flow allowed her to perform movements that would otherwise have been difficult or even harmful.

After a while, Sophia came to understand how she tensed her body. By sometimes experiencing her body as relaxed, she became aware of the difference. She could now work on moving with minimal strain. When we massaged Sophia's feet, it took her half an hour before she could rotate her ankle without tensing her legs, back, chest, and stomach. In a short time, her calf muscles, some of which had been as hard as steel from the tension of overworking, began to loosen. Other calf muscles had deteriorated from being completely unused, and those slowly began to build up. This allowed her to stand more solidly on her feet, but it didn't completely solve her balance problem. At one point, I asked Sophia to stand on one foot. She began to fall over, but

I caught her. Over time, we spent hours doing this before she was able to stand on one foot for even a few seconds. Once she accomplished this, she found it a little easier to stay upright on two feet.

Danny, Vered, and I also worked on other parts of Sophia's body. Her hip joints were very tight, and this restricted her walking a great deal, so I told her to stand on both feet and rotate her pelvis. Although this is a simple motion for most people, Sophia found it nearly impossible. She swung her hips in jerky, angular motions rather than in circles. Vered, who had a lot of experience with this exercise, showed her how to begin by making small circles and gradually increasing the range of movement. She had Sophia tilt her pelvis forward, backward, right, and left. With time, Sophia learned to feel how much she could tilt without falling. Her balance began to improve, and her hip joints became much looser. She began to feel more confident while walking.

Just as Danny, Vered, and I had done, Sophia began to work on herself with an almost fanatic zeal. She exercised for hours every day, and she came to see us three times a week. While she lay on the table, one of us would take her arm or leg and gently stretch it, telling her to imagine that the limb stretched the length of the room, the length of the street, and finally into infinity. We did this with each limb, and she felt as if her body expanded farther every time. As we stretched her limbs, we lengthened the muscles, allowing them to relax. Tense muscles are shorter, and they limit circulation by constricting the blood vessels. This feeling of expansion was relaxing for Sophia, and it made her feel lighter and more open. As she put it, her body seemed to lose its boundaries. The restrictions that tension had imposed on her body seemed to dissolve.

The change in Sophia's concept of her body and its abilities led to a change in her concept of herself. Just as her body expanded and became capable of more and more, so did her sense of herself. In less than half a year, Sophia became an entirely different person. She wanted to learn new things, expand her narrow horizons, and change. She was especially eager to learn whatever she could from us. Sophia was a pleasure to work with. When we showed her an exercise that was difficult at first, she would practice it at home and, two days later, show us that she had mastered it. Our sessions were a mutually beneficial exchange.

Although Sophia didn't exhibit any symptoms of damage to her optic nerve, I thought she might be vulnerable to eye problems since these are common to the multiple sclerosis family of diseases. A person can have an inherent tendency toward a problem without show-ing any symptoms, so rather than wait for this symptom to manifest, I decided to offer preventive therapy; I showed her palming, sunning, and other eye exercises. She got headaches after doing them, but I explained that this was common for someone just beginning to do these exercises; the muscular relaxation makes one more aware of pre-viously unnoticed tension around the eyes. This tension, along with increased stimulation of the optic nerve, was partially responsible for her headaches. The headaches, therefore, were a sign that her nerves needed to be stimulated and relaxed, and that it had been a good idea to give her the eye exercises. I showed Sophia how to massage her head and face to relieve the headaches, but there was a lot of work to do to awaken and heal her degenerated optic nerve. It took eighteen months before Sophia could do eye exercises daily, in comfort.

After only six months, most of Sophia's symptoms had disappeared. She and her husband took walks together every evening, and he was more tired than she at the end of a mile. Only one major symptom remained: Sophia still could feel nothing in her hands and feet. I called Dr. Arkin, an associate of Sophia's neurologist, and he said there was nothing that could be done to restore her sensation. He had studied her case, and the damage was in her central nervous system. "To the best of my knowl-edge," he said, "there has been no case of multiple sclerosis in which sensation has returned, so please just be grateful for what an excellent job you have done." I was not convinced that Dr. Arkin was right. I felt that if anyone deserved health, it was Sophia. She had worked hard on herself, and she was doing everything she could to get well.

I started to rub Sophia's fingers every time she came to see me, put-ting all my love and faith into each massage. I used hand cream to warm her skin and reduce the friction of massage. Each time, I asked her, "Can you feel anything now?" and she answered, "No, not a thing."

Finally, in despair, I called Miriam one evening. I described Sophia's condition, and after asking a few questions Miriam under-stood the whole picture. She asked me, "You know what to do in a case like this, don't you?" "Would I ask you if I knew?" I answered impatiently. Ignoring me, Miriam continued, "It's so simple. All you have to do is tell her to tap her fingers on a table."

I was astonished. It really was simple. Why hadn't I thought of that? I was certain that Sophia would be able to feel with her hands. I didn't understand the effect such an exercise would have, but it was clear to me that stimulating the nerve endings in this way would influence the central nervous system.

Sophia came for her next appointment on a Friday morning, ready to face a hectic day of preparations and then a restful Sabbath. She was surprised when I asked her to sit down at my desk rather than go into the treatment room. Then I sat down beside her. At that moment, my empathy with Sophia was so complete that I experienced a mental union with her.

As Miriam suggested, I told Sophia to tap her fingertips on the desktop. She responded without hesitation, tapping quickly and rhythmically. At first this caused her some pain, but the pain diminished after tapping about 50 times, and then it disappeared. After tapping about 100 times, she began to sense pressure in her fingertips. She continued the tapping, and the pressure also gradually disappeared. After she had tapped about 300 times, she felt only numbness. I was doing the exercise with her and, to my astonishment, it was as if I felt each of her feelings in my own body. By the time we reached 700 taps, there was no pain and no pressure — only a continuous feeling of stimulation. I told Sophia to breathe deeply and relax her shoulders so that we could continue the exercise as long as possible. After tapping 1,000 times, her hands felt as if they were capable of complete, normal sensation.

Then we started to tap the knuckles nearest the fingertips on the desk, and we had the same experience, but it took only half as long to achieve the same results we'd had with the fingertips. We tapped gently at first, slowly increasing the intensity. When the pain came, it was a strong sensation, not numb or distant. Then we repeated the exercise with the middle knuckles with similar results, with an even greater level of sensation, pressure, and pain. Once the process of awakening had begun, it was almost instantaneous.

Finally, we worked on the largest knuckles, where the fingers connect to the hand, and it followed the same progression. First she felt numbness, then pain, then painless pressure, then tingling. We continued by tapping on the table with the wrist bones adjacent to the little finger. By this time, Sophia was able to feel everything she touched, and her hands no longer felt clenched and locked, as they had for months; they actually felt relaxed.

I let Sophia lie down on the table, and I massaged her for a while.

Then I began to test her. With her eyes closed, I put a pen in her hand; she was able to identify it by touch. I gave her a pencil, and she identified it as a pencil, not a pen, because she could feel that it was made of wood. I called Danny and Vered in to share in our triumph. I was so happy that I was in tears. Sophia's was the greatest improvement I had ever seen. For Sophia and me, this was the happiest day of our lives.

For the next few weeks, we used the same exercise to help restore sensation in Sophia's feet. It took longer to accomplish this than with her fingers. Sophia couldn't raise her legs easily, so we assisted her in tapping with her feet. But after three weeks, she began to feel something in her heels. With a lot of exercise and massage, some — though not all — of her feeling was regained.

I called Miriam to tell her about Sophia's success, and she took the news calmly; the results were as she had expected. Then with great excitement, I called Dr. Arkin. He was incredulous and even defensive at first, but soon he was convinced that I was telling the truth. When he saw Sophia a few weeks later, he was amazed. As a result, he began to refer other neurological patients to us.

The doctors at Sophia's hospital had a different reaction. When they saw Sophia's vast improvement, they decided that she'd had a remission after all, and rediagnosed her as having the relapsing-remitting form of multiple sclerosis. They overlooked the fact that no multiple sclerosis patient had ever previously been known to experience remission from a prolonged and total lack of sensation. We are not talking about numbness, which is a sensation in itself, but about a total lack of feeling.

I cannot claim to have a cure for multiple sclerosis, but I can offer the possibility of health for anyone willing to invest the time and effort. Sophia was such a person. She was determined to cure herself, and she succeeded. She thoroughly earned that cure. Sophia had no preconceptions or prejudices; she didn't approach the matter intellectually. She just proceeded with confidence and trust that something would happen. With such an attitude, any disease can be overcome.

Menachem: Up from Despair

A SHORT TIME LATER, Dr. Arkin referred Menachem to us. Menachem owned a restaurant. He'd been hospitalized frequently with multiple sclerosis attacks, and he was overcome with despair. He spent two weeks in the hospital, unable to lie, sit, or stand without feeling dizzy. When he was released, still suffering from dizziness, he went to the hospital's neurology department, where the five neurology specialists were having a meeting. He interrupted them to tell his story, and asked, "Is there anything you can do for me?" They all shook their heads. So Menachem left, but he waited outside the door. As the neurologists left, he asked each of them, one by one, "Can you help me?" Each one repeated, "No, I'm sorry." But Dr. Arkin added, "I know of no cure for multiple sclerosis, but I can give you an unofficial referral to some people who have had some success with it. I am not referring you to these people in my capacity as a doctor; this is strictly off the record." Dr. Arkin was very cautious, and he made it clear that he could promise nothing.

So Menachem came to us as a last resort. I understood Dr. Arkin's pessimism as soon as I started to evaluate Menachem; his legs were so weak that he could barely stand. A muscle test had shown that his leg muscles were almost nonfunctional. His limbs felt very heavy, both to him and to us. Danny commented that the more alive a person is, the lighter his limbs feel — and that this feeling of heaviness is a kind of death. Vered added that this sensation of heaviness has nothing to do with actual weight.

If Menachem merely turned his head to one side, he would lose his balance and fall. He walked like a drunk, swinging his whole body from side to side. He was constantly fatigued, and he simply seemed tired of life. He could see no sense in doing anything; every movement brought with it a bout of dizziness, often accompanied by nausea.

At first, we had no idea what to do. No medical answers had been found. Doctors had tried giving him cortisone, and sometimes vitamin B12, but these had not succeeded in alleviating any of his symptoms. Even during his remissions, Menachem's dizziness worsened every day.

Menachem's wife had left him because of his illness, and his children came to see him only occasionally. He had been forced to lease out his restaurant because he couldn't run it by himself. He was about to sell his house and go live with his parents; he'd only delayed doing so because he didn't have the physical or emotional strength to put his house on the market.

During our first meeting with Menachem, I told him that we expected him to do a number of exercises. I could feel his reluctance to doing anything; it wasn't only the strain and discomfort that any action caused him, it was also that his body needed a lot of rest. We decided to see Menachem three times a week.

The first thing I did with Menachem was to slowly, gently move each of his limbs to encourage circulation. We also went to work on his eye problems; his optic nerve had degenerated, and his vision was blurred. Palming helped a great deal; not only did it give his eyes some relief, but through resting his eyes he was able to relax his whole body. He became aware of a feeling that something was constantly choking him from within, emotionally and physically, and this feeling was released when he palmed.

After only two weeks, Menachem's walking began to show signs of improvement. We had instructed him to rotate his feet several hundred times a day, and as a result his calves were stronger. Feeling more relaxed increased his confidence, and his constant fear of falling was alleviated. But he still limped, and it was difficult for him to raise his legs.

During our seventh session, Menachem said, "I'm starting to get better. I'm still dizzy and I'm still limping, but I feel better inside. I feel like I want to do things." He told me that, the day before, he had gone to his restaurant and asked the people who were leasing it to let him do some work there. He had felt dizzy, but he worked for two hours. "I'm tired of staying in bed," he confided. This improvement touched me deeply. I felt a change in his state of mind, and I believed that he was going to succeed in his quest for improvement.

Menachem still had ups and downs. At one session, he told Vered that he didn't know how he could continue to live with constant dizziness. But his new hope could meet that despair. It was during that session with Vered, while she massaged the back of his head, that he experienced his first temporary relief from dizziness. Though this reprieve only lasted a few hours, it was a sign that the condition could be relieved.

Miriam had once told me that she'd suffered from severe headaches for many years. One headache had been so extreme that she couldn't do anything. In the midst of it, she lay down on the floor and began to slowly move her head from side to side. At first the pain increased even more, and she felt as if her whole body would explode, but she continued to rotate her head while massaging her scalp. Within thirty minutes, the headache passed, and she never had another one. This is like piling blankets on a patient with a high fever to help her "sweat out" the fever; the symptom is encouraged to reach a peak level so that it can pass more quickly. This is in the spirit of the fundamental principle of homeopathy: like treats like. It occurred to me that Menachem's problem might be treated in a similar way.

One day, after two and a half months of working with Menachem, he arrived at our office suffering as much as ever from dizziness. I asked him to stand in front of the window and rotate his head from side to side. "I can't possibly do that," he protested. "I'm dizzy enough as it is." But I insisted, and for some reason he trusted me enough to try it. He turned his head from left to right and back again once, and he felt nauseated. He tried again and grew even sicker, with a suffocating sensation in his solar plexus. On the third try, he thought he would vomit; on the fourth try, he did. Then his face turned a pale yellow-green, and he said, "I'm going to faint." His body was cold and moist, so I helped him onto the table and rubbed him with oil to warm him. I massaged him until he was warm again, the nausea had passed, and his skin was rosy.

We went out onto the porch and tried again. He felt weak and sick, but this time he was able to turn his head seven times before he became pale and chilled. Then he vomited again. I took him back to the table for another massage.

We did this a third time with the same results. I could hardly believe that either of us was willing to continue, but somehow we both felt that we were doing the right thing. After the fourth try, Menachem began to have less trouble with the exercise. His circulation was becoming better, and it created a more even distribution of blood between his head and his body.

We repeated the exercise ten times! Each time, it seemed to affect him a little less. The tenth time, I led him to the porch and he was able to move his head thirty times in each direction. After that, he said, "I'm not dizzy and I don't feel sick, but I'm very weak and tired." We agreed that this was enough for one day. I massaged him again, instructed him not to eat anything for the rest of the day, and called a cab to take him home.

Menachem began to do this exercise daily. The next day, he was able to rotate his head two hundred times without becoming dizzy. From that time on, he improved dramatically. He could walk down the street and turn his head from side to side to look at the store windows. He could ride a bicycle for half an hour and could even jog a little.

Having been granted relief from his worst problem, Menachem began to get in touch with other aspects of his illness. He could now feel how weak and stiff his movements were, and how imbalanced his standing and walking. This new awareness changed Menachem's whole approach to life. No longer a hopeless victim of a mysterious ailment, he could now look at the cause of his problems and make an effort to change.

Working with Menachem taught me much about the importance of restoring the center of movement when treating multiple sclerosis. After we had helped him overcome his dizziness and regain his balance, we had to help him restructure his entire habitual pattern of movement, especially walking, and help him rebuild the muscles in his legs and feet.

Menachem's center of movement was in the back of his head where it joins the neck, making it difficult for him to breathe deeply. This was indicated by the tension there, and by the fact that he threw his entire weight on his toes when he walked. I asked him to stand up straight and keep his feet parallel when he stood or walked, and to concentrate on his body's true center, just below the navel. I instructed him to breathe deeply into his abdomen to increase his awareness of that area so that he could begin to refocus his center of movement there, where it belonged. This exercise of "centering" helps people become aware of where the impetus behind a movement comes from. This is not esoteric knowledge; anyone who pays attention to his or her body can learn to center.

As Menachem breathed into his abdomen, a sensation of lightness flowed through him. I placed my hands on his abdomen and asked him to visualize his back relaxing and growing wider and longer. When I did this, Menachem experienced a great release of his neck tension and could move his neck from side to side with no restriction — farther than he had ever been able to before. As he continued moving his head from side to side — visualizing his back growing wider and stronger, his neck lengthening, the top of his head going up to the sky, and his energy flowing from his center — Menachem's thoracic vertebrae began to make popping sounds, even though I wasn't touching them. This is a sign that his spine was lengthening and relaxing.

We then tried to incorporate this new awareness into Menachem's walking. His inclination was to return to his unbalanced, constricted walk. I coached him, reminding him to concentrate on his center and feel his back expanding, his shoulders extending, and his neck lengthening. I then asked him to sit and then rise without using his arms to help him. This was difficult for someone whose leg muscles were so tight as to be nearly paralyzed. He had come to the point where he no longer sat down; he just collapsed into a chair, then used his arms to push himself up. Stretching and exercising his thigh muscles, and maintaining an awareness of his abdominal center as the focal point of movement, eventually enabled Menachem to sit and rise in a coordinated, relaxed way.

My Lecture to the Multiple Sclerosis Society

MANY YEARS LATER, I was invited to speak at a conference of the Multiple Sclerosis Society in British Columbia, Canada. I wanted to give them a fresh perspective on their condition, and to lead them in some exercises that could help them. Nearly 300 people with multiple sclerosis attended my lecture. It was a challenge to address the issues that were of interest to all the participants, since people with multiple sclerosis tend to suffer from varied symptoms, with different expressions. Nevertheless, in spite of their different symptoms and their different lives, there were a few things they all had in common.

My advice to them was different than what they were used to hearing. People suffering from multiple sclerosis are usually advised to use a cane if they don't walk well, then to use crutches or walkers and finally wheelchairs as they lose strength and balance. I said the opposite: If you don't walk well, don't use a cane unless you fall frequently and might break your bones. If you do use a cane, crutches, or walkers, find every opportunity to walk without them. If you've been in a wheelchair for a short time, do all you can to get out of it as soon as possible. Those devices are addictive; once you get used to them, your self-image builds around them, and sooner or later you can't do without them. As you grow accustomed to using these devices, you subconsciously feel that you have no other choice. But there's much more to the problem than that. Sitting in a wheelchair decreases your circulation and weakens your muscles. If you start using a wheelchair out of convenience when you still have a choice about whether to use it, you will eventually become too weak to do without it. I had the sense that my audience agreed. I also got the impression that most of them felt they had started using their canes too early.

People who suffer from multiple sclerosis are often more fatigued than most other people. While others can get some rest when they're tired, and overcome their fatigue quickly, people with multiple sclerosis may find that their fatigue stays with them for days or weeks. This, I found, was another point that the group had in common: If you have multiple sclerosis, you have to address your fatigue immediately. No matter what you have to do in life, I told them, the moment you feel fatigue you should rest; it's an acknowledgment of the specific disability you have. I stressed the fact that there's a difference between acknowledging a disability and succumbing to it. To be more specific, there's a difference between working constantly on your mobility and resting when you need to, and giving in to the disability.

I then shared with the audience my favorite relaxation exercise:

Multiple Sclerosis Exercise: Breathing Relaxation

Lie down on your back. Bend your knees if you can do that easily, placing your feet on the ground or mat. If this is not possible, rest your legs on two or three pillows. Now breathe deeply, but not forcibly, through your nose and visualize your body expanding when you inhale, and shrinking when you exhale. Breathe deeply again, and visualize the spaces between your vertebrae increasing. Relax and breathe deeply as you imagine that your shoulders are growing distant from one another and that your neck is lengthening. Spend three to five minutes with this exercise. Here's another of my favorite breathing relaxations: Lying on your back, inhale, exhale, remain without air to the count of thirty, then inhale slowly and deeply. Repeat this three times.

Pointers for Exercising

I TOLD THE GROUP that they might work on their bodies and not overcome all their symptoms. I added that they might sometimes find that, even when doing their best, their body isn't getting better — or perhaps it even gets worse. But I added that it is my experience that, in most cases, we can prevent deterioration by learning the ins and outs of our bodies. I find that working to increase mobility and overcome other symptoms is better than any positive affirmation; it is the actual physical action that can help us avoid the hazards of depression, stay optimistic and positive, and maintain a healthy approach. If you can get even a little bit better, it is worth the effort. If you can slow your deterioration, you're working for a good cause.

I then led the group in doing the exercise for the ring muscles that control elimination (see chapter 10, "Do the Locomotive"). It is an important exercise for those who have lost bladder control and those who have partial control. Because it influences the autonomic nervous system, even people who don't have urinary problems but are under stress can benefit from this exercise. Most people in the group had a great sense of relaxation after practicing it.

I explained to the audience the principle of building strength from their base: If your toes are weak, the ankle muscles have to tense up to stabilize the foot. The knee then becomes stiff to adjust to the stiffness of the ankle. The hip joint becomes stiff to adjust to the stiffness of the knees. Consequently, the back and neck tighten up, too. Therefore, strengthening the toes can help loosen the ankles and relieve stiffness in the whole body.

I then guided them in a couple of exercises for the toes and ankles:

Multiple Sclerosis Exercise: Strengthening Toes and Loosening Ankles

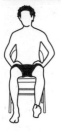

While sitting on a chair with your feet on the floor, use your toes to move your feet forward, inch by inch.

Still seated on the chair, keep your heel down and raise the front of your foot up from the floor; alternate between left and right.

Building Strong Feet and Calves

I THEN TOLD THE GROUP that working on the toes and feet has another important benefit: Building up strong feet and calves provides better stability, which will aid in keeping your balance. If you sit in a wheelchair and cannot walk, working on your lower body in any way possible can help stabilize your upper body to some extent.

I instructed those in the group who were ambulatory to stand up and massage one foot by rolling a tennis ball under it. (Those who weren't able to stand up either rolled a tennis ball under their foot while sitting, or imagined that they were doing so if they couldn't physically do it.) Here is the exercise we did:

Multiple Sclerosis Exercise: Tennis-Ball Foot Massage

Place a tennis ball on the floor underneath one foot. Putting pressure on the ball, move your foot from side to side, letting the ball massage underneath your toes, your arch, and then your heel. Now mentally divide the foot lengthwise into three portions, and roll the tennis ball from the big toe to the heel and back, from the middle toes to the heel and back, and from the little toe to the heel and back.

When the process was finished, those who'd participated found themselves standing with much more confidence and less fear of falling.

Fine Control of Movement

FINE CONTROL OF MOVEMENT was the group's main interest. I explained that when we are born, we do not have the fine control over movement that we eventually achieve. Our nerves and our myelin sheath develop as we build our capability to refine our movements. Then, in cases of multiple sclerosis, people lose the capability for fine movement, and at the same time the myelin sheath deteriorates. It seemed that my listeners could all relate to that, whether they were wheelchair-bound or had minimal symptoms. I continued that line of thought and suggested that, in my experience, working on building up refined movement seems to have a positive impact on the nervous system; perhaps it rebuilds myelin.

I told the group my opinion, based on my extensive work with multiple sclerosis: that everyone could get better, as long as they were attentive and well aware of their restrictions. If one's restriction is fatigue, one needs to be aware of it, have a sense of when it is coming, and rest. If the restriction is a lack of will to move resulting from depression, one needs to immediately start using gentle, subtle movement exercises to reduce the feeling of hopelessness. Movement that leads to a change of pattern — movement that is out of the ordinary for us — is the kind of movement that will help strengthen the central nervous system.

It is possible to improve one's level of fine control, but people can benefit quickly from learning the level of control that is available to them, which they may not be aware of. I led the group through the following exercises to help them assess their present level of fine control:

Multiple Sclerosis Exercise: Opening and Closing the Hand

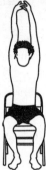

Open and close your hands extremely slowly, feeling every part of the motion. Stop and visualize the movement, then try it again. The movement will probably feel smoother the second time through, even if you suffer from a tremor.

Now interlace the fingers of both hands and stretch your arms up, with your palms facing the ceiling.

Repeat the exercise of slowly opening and closing your hand.

With this exercise, you can pay attention to the control of your hand and, subtly, to where the control has been lost. Even if your movement feels perfectly good or normal to you, you may find some parts unsmooth or stiff, while other parts are smoother. With enough repetition, visualization, and careful attention, you can improve your ability to open and close your hand smoothly.

Multiple Sclerosis Exercise: Turning the Head

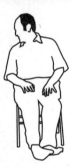

Most people tend to tense their necks when they move their feet, and vice versa. The purpose of this exercise is to isolate the feet and neck from each other in order to create better control and coordination.

Move your head from side to side. If possible, rotate your feet in the opposite direction. If you can't move your feet, imagine that your feet are rotating in the opposite direction from your head. This exercise is a challenge to most everyone I know, whether or not their movement is limited.

Beyond Medication

FINALLY, I addressed the subject of medication. Many people with multiple sclerosis are taking medication, and many will take other medications as they are developed over the years. I told them that, in my opinion, practicing movement, as I had just taught them to do, would always be a better tool for improving their health.

I told the audience several success stories from among my multiple sclerosis patients. As I described one patient after another — their struggles and their achievements — I knew that my audience suddenly felt, at least for a little while, that they had energy to give to themselves. At the completion of the lecture and exercises, I could sense optimism in the group.

Following are two more of the stories I told them about patients whose lives were improved by self-healing movement.

Ruth: Increasing Mobility and Stability

RUTH MET ME for sessions whenever I visited London. Because of multiple sclerosis, she walked with a limp and had little stability. We used the following eye exercise to help her reduce the instability:

Multiple Sclerosis Exercise: Balancing the Eyes

Tape a small piece of paper (about 2 inches long by 1 1/2 inches wide) to the bridge of your nose with the longer direction vertical. Now, looking straight ahead, wave your hands at the sides of your head so that each eye can see one hand.

The purpose of this exercise is to encourage the brain to balance the use of the eyes. It is especially important if you have lost vision because of multiple sclerosis. I recommend practicing this exercise for seven minutes a day.

I also had Ruth walk backward. (See page 122, "Walk Sideways or Backward.") This exercise temporarily improved her balance.

Ruth's mobility was stable for several years until one winter, during which time she was able to walk very little because of the weather and other stressors. When she started to walk again, she was much weaker.

Multiple Sclerosis in Cold and Hot Weather

MUSCLES WEAKENED by multiple sclerosis cannot afford to be immobile for a long period of time. The cost of this lost time can be loss of mobility. Rainy or snowy winters can make it difficult or impossible for a person with a poor gait to go out; in such cases, it's important to find ways to work on oneself indoors.

Hot summers aren't any better. The majority of multiple sclerosis patients have much poorer mobility during hot summers. On hot summer days, I suggest taking five cold showers or baths a day. If you have multiple sclerosis, make sure that every two hours you are under a cold shower (three to four minutes) or in a cold bath (four to five minutes). If you're not able to do that, at least put an ice pack on your neck for seven to ten minutes every two hours. If you allow your body to heat up, you could be subject to attacks of multiple sclerosis, and that could decrease your mobility. Many people gain mobility when they cool themselves; it is the frequency of cooling that makes a difference. I can't emphasize it enough: Don't ignore your disease. Treat it while working on living a normal life. Give your body what it needs to sustain itself, and your life will be more normal with time.

Getting Out of the Wheelchair

OVER THE YEARS, I saw Ruth for several sessions every time I visited London. However, I didn't see her during the winter that led to her deterioration. Years later, Ruth had a session with me in San Francisco. She was in a wheelchair and unable to bend her knees. I knew that her inability to bend her knees wasn't a result of the neurological damage of multiple sclerosis; it had to do with being confined to a wheelchair. True, it was the multiple sclerosis that got her in the wheelchair in the first place, but some of the muscles that had worked well before she started using the wheelchair were now tight and frozen. More than half of the problems related to multiple sclerosis, in my experience, are secondary to the disease, and they can be overcome.

I used deep tissue massage on Ruth's legs, leaving her legs with black and blue marks. We joked about how close the nearest police station was. After the massage, Ruth was able to bend her legs. Then I put her in a cold bath, which she really didn't enjoy, for fifteen minutes. At first she sat in the bathtub protesting and singing loudly, but drinking hot tea while sitting in the cold water made her feel a little better.

Next I took Ruth to the beach in her wheelchair, where she was able to walk several yards and then crawl on the sand. She was smiling and her eyes sparkled with the joy of feeling so mobile again.

Ruth returned to England with renewed enthusiasm. She was able to stay out of her wheelchair most of the day. She also crawled for forty minutes a day and walked for at least ten minutes a day. Although she spent most of the day sitting, she was able to move from one position to another and maintain different sitting postures during the day. Every step forward can uplift the spirit.

Shannon: Regaining Eyesight Damaged by Multiple Sclerosis

SHANNON WAS A beautiful young woman who'd had a severe, paralyzing attack of multiple sclerosis following surgery. It is not uncommon for attacks of multiple sclerosis to be triggered by shock or trauma; surgery may, indeed, qualify as a physical trauma to the body. When Shannon was diagnosed with progressive multiple sclerosis, one of her physicians told her parents that she would soon be either institutionalized or dead. Her parents massaged her, got her out of bed, and worked with her using movement and massage until she was able to walk. Eventually, she was able to travel from Pennsylvania to San Francisco on her own to see me for two weeks of intensive sessions.

One of Shannon's eyes was nearly blinded by the attack of multiple sclerosis. Her other eye had always been a "lazy eye," and her brain didn't engage with it. Consequently, she couldn't read or drive, and she felt visually disoriented. I taught her the palming exercise to relax her eyes, but she hated it; she couldn't feel relaxed enough to do it.

Shannon was a massage therapist. One time, when I needed a massage myself after extensive dental work, she gave me a massage. I took advantage of the opportunity and asked her to put her hands over my eyes and palm them. I'm accustomed to palming on my own, but when someone palms my eyes they relax even better.

Shannon had no adverse relationship with my eyes — only with her own. When her hands rested on my eyes, she felt the way my eyes were relaxing and realized that palming would be useful to her. She still hated to palm, so when she returned home, she got her parents to palm her eyes. Consequently, her eyes got better.

Because Shannon's formerly strong right eye was nearly blinded by the multiple sclerosis attack, she no longer used it. Although her brain didn't engage well with her lazy left eye, it now engaged even less with her right eye. I therefore had to teach her to break that pattern and learn to use the two eyes together. I instructed her to tape a small piece of paper (about $1\frac{1}{2}$ inches long by 1 inch wide) on the bridge of her nose to separate the visual fields of both eyes. I asked her to look straight ahead with the damaged right eye while waving her hand in front of the lazy left eye. The purpose of this exercise was to stimulate her right eye to see, while sending a message to her brain that her left eye needed to be engaged simultaneously. Somehow, when she used both eyes at the same time in this way, she was able to read with her left eye, which had been lazy all her life. Optometrists and ophthalmologists usually believe that a lazy eye cannot recover after the age of eight or nine. Until that age, they would exercise a lazy eye and patch the other one, but after that age they'd drop the program. Shannon managed to regain use of her lazy eye at the age of twenty-two. Her vision improved to 20/50 in that left eye — 20/20 with correction — and she developed the ability to read and drive while depending on it. Shannon's mobility and confidence increased, and her level of fatigue decreased. She was able to attend my intensive practitioner training classes, which she used to benefit herself and many others.

There are many exercises for multiple sclerosis, but the most important factor is to maintain confidence that improvement can happen. You will hear many opinions to the contrary. Regardless of those, if you have multiple sclerosis, try to move forward, reconstruct your myelin sheath, and regain function. I hope that you will find energy to give to yourself, for it is when we deplete ourselves of our own energy that we don't search for answers.

CHAPTER 12

BREATHING, VISUALIZATION, AND BODY AWARENESS

Visualization is a powerful tool for improving the body's function. It can help increase circulation, improve movement, reduce and eliminate inflammation, reduce pain, and enhance the senses of vision, hearing, and touch. Visualization unveils our subconscious thoughts regarding the functioning of our bodies, and consciously corrects that functioning. In a circular process of improvement, visualization enhances one's awareness of one's body, and as one's awareness improves, one's visualizations become more effective.

Mr. Solano: Breathing Away Minor Back Pain and Headaches

MR. SOLANO heard me lecture at the Vegetarian Society. He had no serious malady, but he wanted to use his minor, ordinary problems as a way to learn about himself. A handsome man in his late forties, Mr. Solano told me that he had a minor back problem and was often tired. He also had occasional headaches. He was a very open-minded, inquisitive man.

Mr. Solano had developed some tightness in his lower back as a result of poor posture and poor walking habits. Instead of putting his weight equally on each foot and equally on each part of the feet, he tended to land heavily on his right heel, which created pressure in his lower back. He wasn't especially concerned about his spine problem becoming more serious, but he felt that if he could learn to relax his back he would be able to relax his whole body, and as a result eliminate his headaches.

Not surprisingly, the treatment we found most effective for Mr. Solano was to regulate and deepen his breathing. Shallow breathing causes constriction of every part of the body. With less oxygen coming in, all functioning becomes more difficult; one's energy level drops, and fatigue sets in. The heart is particularly affected, since the working of the lungs and heart are so closely connected.

If there is more oxygen in the body because of deeper breathing, the heart doesn't have to strain to pump blood to the rest of the body. Every cell in the body requires fresh oxygen as its fuel, and this is carried to each cell by the flow of blood. Veins carry deoxygenated blood into the heart, and the heart pumps it into the lungs, where it is enriched with oxygen. The blood then returns to the heart, which pumps it through the arteries to the cells. If you do not breathe deeply enough to take in sufficient oxygen, the blood will leave the lungs without enough oxygen to adequately nourish the cells. The cells will then need to send the blood back for oxygen more frequently, requiring the heart to pump more than would be necessary if proper breathing had supplied enough oxygen to the lungs in the first place. With chronic shallow breathing, the cells are not adequately nourished, and one begins to feel fatigued. After a while, the cells become accustomed to this and don't even demand more oxygen. Fatigue, low energy, depression, and many common problems become a way of life. We no longer recognize them as problems, but they leave us more vulnerable to illness.

The way we breathe has an effect on our emotional lives. Fear, anger, and other negative emotions lose some of their impact when we breathe deeply, slowly, and regularly. Deep breathing brings with it a sense of peace and harmony. Breath is life, and the more slowly and deeply you breathe the more alive you are.

I asked Mr. Solano to inhale and hold his breath for a count of sixty, then exhale and count to sixty before inhaling again, and to repeat this exercise ten times in a relaxed manner akin to meditation. It took him several weeks to work up to a count of sixty. To do this, we had to use massage and exercise on his diaphragm, chest, and abdominal muscles, all of which are involved in deep breathing. This exercise encourages the patient to enjoy as fully as possible the benefits of oxygen. It creates a feeling in the body quite different from that created by rapid, shallow breathing.

I asked Mr. Solano to visualize his breath as a breeze blowing down into his abdomen, then up his spine and into the back of his neck. I also asked him to describe what his breath sounded like, to encourage him to really listen to the sound and to experience deep relaxation. As Mr. Solano lay there listening to his breath, he suddenly got quite cold. It was 90 degrees Fahrenheit — a warm summer afternoon — yet he was trembling. We were both startled, and Mr. Solano asked me why he was feeling so cold. I thought for a while, and the answer came: "You must be deeply relaxed." He responded, still shivering, "Yes, I am. In fact, I feel more relaxed and comfortable than ever." I have since observed that this commonly occurs during full relaxation.

From that time on, Mr. Solano felt increasingly relaxed and expansive from within. He became so relaxed, in fact, that he set a new standard of relaxation for me. He stood evenly balanced on both feet. The tension that had controlled his mind and body for thirty years, which had brought on headaches, backaches, and a perpetual state of impatience and frustration, completely dissolved. Simple breathing exercises practiced for less than a month cured him of all these problems, and his general attitude about himself improved immensely.

Viva: Relief of Anemia through Improved Circulation

AT ABOUT THE SAME TIME, I began to work with a woman named Viva, who was suffering from a type of anemia in which her body's supply of red blood cells had become depleted. (This is only one of many types of anemia, but it is one of the most common.) Red blood cells are produced in the marrow of certain bones, such as the sternum, vertebrae, and others. Through movement, breathing, and bodywork, we can improve circulation and possibly the production of red blood cells in the bone marrow.

Viva was a short, thin woman whose face was pale from lack of circulation. The skin on her palms and the soles of her feet was tough and rigid, and she suffered from eczema. She was constantly fatigued, and when she came to my office at the Vegetarian Society, she looked exhausted.

Viva was in her mid-thirties, the wife of a bus driver and the mother of two small children. Her parents were still so deeply involved in her life that she didn't know how to free herself from their influence. Viva felt completely oppressed by her circumstances. She felt that she had no control of her life or her decisions.

Physicians tend to view anemia solely in terms of blood chemistry and treat it accordingly, but I think it should be viewed in terms of circulation. Severely inadequate circulation, I believe, leads to iron deficiency. I knew that stimulating Viva's circulation would stimulate the organs responsible for the production of red blood cells.

I had two main objectives in my treatment of Viva. First, I wanted to create good, strong circulation throughout her body. Second, I wanted to strengthen and relax her exhausted body. I told Viva to take alternating hot and cold showers. Warm water brings blood circulation to the surface, relaxing the muscles, and cold water sends the blood deeper into the body's tissues, stimulating the internal organs and making the blood run faster to maintain the body's warmth. By relaxing her hip joints and shoulders with gentle exercise, and by massaging her hands and feet, we increased her circulation by drawing blood into her extremities, thus making it flow strongly throughout her entire body. This, along with the application of a moisturizing cream, helped relieve her eczema as well.

I also taught Viva how to breathe deeply, which is extremely helpful to circulation, enriching the blood with oxygen. We used very few other movements at first. It was more helpful for her to simply lie and breathe. I was careful that she did not expend effort in breathing, for even breathing was an exertion for her; she needed to learn to breathe without straining.

Then we began to work with small movements to reduce the stiffness in Viva's muscles and joints, a condition that often accompanies anemia. I taught her to rub her hands together and then to rub her feet together while holding onto her calves. This was particularly difficult for her, and she grew tired almost immediately. In order to rub her feet together, she used her back, shoulders, and abdomen with great effort. When she learned to relax the muscles that weren't needed for this movement, this exercise became very helpful for her, and she would do it continually until her feet became warm.

I also massaged Viva's entire body, especially her cold, pale hands and feet. Her hands had a greenish tint and her feet were almost orange, but after massage both were a normal pinkish color. I worked a lot on her chest. Negative emotions are often stored in the muscles of the chest.

I showed Viva several ways to massage her hands. First, she would rub her hands together about one hundred times. Then she would rub only the fingertips against each other, and then only the palms, in circular motions. The most effective variation was "hand washing," in which she would rub her hands and fingers together as if lathering them with soap. This motion ensures that each part of the hand is massaged and stimulated.

These simple exercises were difficult for Viva at first, not only because of her physical weakness, but also because they released so much emotion. After each of our early sessions together, Viva left feeling exhausted. She had a lot of difficulty knowing how much she could do physically, as well as knowing what her limits were and when she needed to rest.

Consequently, the next step was to teach Viva relaxation exercises. I instructed her to imagine her body as very heavy, then as very light. I had her picture her blood pouring through her veins, flowing from her head down through her neck. As it reached her chest, she could feel the emotional tension slowly dissolve. She visualized blood flowing through the muscles of her back, her solar plexus, the muscles and organs of her abdominal cavity, then into her pelvis, down her legs, and into her feet. She would spend at least five minutes imagining blood circulating through her feet, imagining each toe growing warm, before visualizing the blood going back up her legs and through the rest of her body until it reached into her hands.

I asked Viva to feel the connection between the toes of her left foot and the fingers of her left hand. By doing so, she encouraged the neurological communication between these two areas. This feeling of interconnectedness increases one's ability to influence the body's functioning, which in turn produces more circulation and vitality.

Gradually, Viva began to overcome her fatigue. After two months of treatment, both our sessions and her solo exercises became a little easier for her. Still, she complained that she frequently felt exhausted. I asked her, "Why don't you do the relaxation exercises each time you feel exhausted?" "I didn't know I was supposed to," she replied. "I thought they were for the exercise period." "Why don't you listen to your body," I asked, "and not just do what you think you are supposed to?" Viva was silent.

After this, whenever Viva felt fatigued she did her relaxation exercises, even if briefly, and then returned to whatever she'd been doing, feeling refreshed. After a few more months, her fatigue disappeared and her hands and feet were warm all the time. I knew then that she was cured from anemia, and her blood tests confirmed this. She felt and acted as if she had come back to life. This whole process took five months.

In the final analysis, most physical problems are in some way related to poor circulation. We work on strengthening the circulation of every patient who comes to us. While good circulation alone might not bring about a cure, no cure is really possible without it.

Dvora: Restoration of Inner Strength

DVORA WAS AN Orthodox Jewish woman in her early forties who had undergone eleven operations for a serious hernia condition; the extreme weakness of her abdominal muscles was hereditary. Her family and community imposed numerous demands on her, which she met with much hardship. Having to observe the many religious strictures was a burden to her, and her slow walk and stooped posture reflected this. Her husband was a self-centered, demanding man who asked a lot more of her than he was willing to give back. He treated her more like a servant than a life companion.

Dvora's shoulders were stiff and tense, and this tension worked its way into every muscle of her body. Though she believed devoutly in her religion, living with so many restrictions left scars of anger and resentment in both her body and her personality. She was a compassionate, generous woman, receptive to new ideas and open to other people. She took care of her family, including her mentally unstable brother, and of everyone and everything around her. She also cared for herself, which was why she came to us despite her husband's scorn.

When I first saw Dvora, it was obvious that she needed to make some major changes in her life. She had lost her inner source of strength in a life of catering to the needs of others. She needed to find her strength again, and to build a life around it. The expression on her face when she walked into my office left a strong impression on me: Her dark eyes were warm and vital, and I saw a compassionate, tender soul hidden behind a tough, aggressive look that had become habitual through years of conflict.

I began by teaching Dvora how to breathe well. This first exercise was very important; lack of oxygen was one reason she always felt so weighted down. Her breathing was shallow and rapid. I taught her to concentrate on her breathing, first by counting the length of each exhalation and inhalation to achieve longer, deeper breaths, then by consciously expanding her abdomen as she breathed. This helped her relax and feel lighter, and it also strengthened her abdominal muscles. After 100 slow, deep breaths, she felt relaxed and certain that she would get better, both physically and mentally.

I explained to Dvora that we would strengthen all the muscles of her abdomen so that the muscles around her intestines would not rupture again. Her muscles were weak and degenerated, but I was sure that she would make whatever effort she needed to improve. The expression on her face had already softened; it now expressed her whole loving soul. She reminded me of my grandmother, who was for me the personification of selfless love, and of Miriam, who led me to eyesight.

After the breathing exercise, I massaged Dvora's abdomen, and the muscles responded immediately. The tighter ones became looser, and the weaker, dead-feeling ones became firmer. Next, I put one hand on her abdomen and the other on her lower back and told Dvora to visualize my two hands meeting inside her abdomen. I told her to imagine that my hands, which were opening, warming, and loosening the muscles of her abdomen and back, were doing the same to her internal muscles, relaxing the entire abdominal cavity. Then I taught her to massage her own abdomen; while she lacked sensitivity, she was able to relax the muscles a little. She breathed more deeply, and she felt great relief by the time she left.

During our next session, while massaging and relaxing Dvora, I gave her a third exercise. Normally, she would just drag her heavy legs while walking, letting her abdominal and lower back muscles contract and do all the work. In fact, she tended to use her entire body to perform any motion, exerting far more effort than was necessary. This kept her body tense and weak. I asked her to consciously direct her legs to work for themselves. She, of course, had a deep resistance to changing her habits. Through deep breathing and constantly reminding herself to use only her legs for walking (or whatever specific muscles were needed for any particular movement), she was able to do this sometimes during our sessions and her exercise periods. My goal was to make correct, effortless movement become automatic for Dvora.

Dvora's husband opposed her treatment with me and refused to support it, so she took a part-time job to cover the expense of the treatment. She said that she thanked God that she could see me while her husband was at work to avoid arguing with him about it. Meanwhile, she was making significant improvements. Her hernia pains recurred occasionally, but the visualization exercise, in which she would imagine my hands going through her abdomen and her back and meeting inside, nearly always relieved the pain. Within three months, her body became much stronger, particularly her abdominal muscles. But she still felt weighed down emotionally. Her daughter, who was nine years old and still wetting the bed, was affected by her mother's suffering and by the problems between her parents.

One day, Dvora came to our center smiling and cheerful, ready to begin our work. She had done her homework, and it was clear to both of us that she had improved greatly. I asked her to breathe deeply and, after a few warm-up exercises and some massage, I lifted one of her legs off the massage table and asked her to feel its heaviness as I held it. Then I set it down and asked her to imagine that I was lifting it again. Even imagining me lifting her leg made her feel 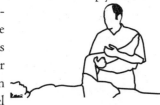 how hard it was to just relax and allow it to be lifted. She grew flushed and nauseated, as if she were straining to lift the leg herself.

Then I asked her to lift the leg; she found this easier than the visualization, as she could use her abdominal muscles to assist the leg. In actually performing the motion, she reverted to her old ways, allowing other muscles to work for her legs, but in visualization she couldn't. She was so dependent on her abdomen, back, and pelvis to help her move the leg that the image of lifting it by its own power overwhelmed her. I tried once again to get her to visualize letting the leg lift itself, and once more she grew flushed and nauseated. When I asked her to imagine lifting both legs together, she actually passed out for a moment.

This experience was overwhelming for Dvora. For the first time, she fully experienced the effects of tension, and she saw clearly that her tension was caused by the way she used her body. She realized what she had to do, and she decided to do it. She left my office that day feeling heavy and a little sick, but with a deep sense of challenge and self-confidence.

After that, Dvora was never the same. From then on, she was able to cope with all of her physical problems; she found imagery to be her most useful tool. She improved the way she did her exercises, and she reached the point where she could raise and lower both legs, together or separately, with little or no effort. One specific visualization brought her the most profound sense of release: She would visualize herself lying on her back and lifting her feet until they stretched behind her head, then rolling forward until her hands touched her toes. She couldn't actually perform these motions, but imagining them helped her immensely.

Dvora began working on herself with the same devotion that she showed her family and her Jewish faith. She grew stronger and felt lighter in body and spirit, and her life changed completely. Her relationship with her husband began to improve — at least from her viewpoint — as she learned to stand up for herself. Her daughter's and brother's problems became a priority, as she was now capable of handling them without harming herself.

It was wonderful to see Dvora blossom in the middle of her life. Her progress was rapid once she realized what she had been doing wrong. By releasing destructive tensions and learning to relax, she had the energy to rebuild herself; her muscles grew stronger all the time until she was completely cured.

Up until then, Dvora had been offered only symptomatic treatment for a deep-rooted problem. Only her ruptured muscles had been dealt with, and not the emotional and physiological pressures that caused the damage. Doctors had been able to fuse the torn muscles surgically, but they couldn't prevent recurrent ruptures. Addressing only effects and not causes is at best unsatisfactory, and can actually be dangerous. When Dvora learned to heal her body at its deepest, most basic level, she not only learned to treat her hernia problem, but she gained the capacity to prevent future recurrences.

Naomi: The Power of Visualization

AFTER THREE MONTHS of working with Naomi, whose story I told in chapter 9 (Back Problems), I decided it was time for us to begin strengthening her legs, abdomen, and lower back. The first exercise I gave her was to raise both legs together while lying on her back. She could barely lift even one leg without a great deal of effort. I told her to imagine that her leg was very heavy and short — short because muscles shorten as they contract. As she practiced this imagery and tried to lift one leg, her lower back tensed and she felt that she could hardly breathe. Next I told her to imagine that the leg was normal in size and in weight. As she did this, her back relaxed and her breathing returned to normal. Then I told her to imagine that the leg had grown longer and was as light as a cloud. When she did this, the muscles of her back relaxed completely, and her back lay almost flat against the table.

This visualization exercise helped Naomi feel the connection between her legs and her back; after doing it, she was able to lift her leg without over-recruiting her back muscles. This gave her a great deal of relief. After we did this with the other leg, I asked Naomi to visualize lifting both her legs up and down twenty times. A severe pain developed in her forehead, so I massaged it to relieve the pain. Gradually, she could not only visualize lifting both legs, but she was able to actually lift them successfully.

Visualization has become essential to our therapeutic approach. I have found it to be beneficial to every part of the body. For certain individuals, visualization has been the key to solving their physical problems. Imagery is important because it helps us recognize our unconscious feelings and conceptions about how our bodies function. Sometimes change can come about through awareness alone, but it generally takes time and work. Naomi had not realized that she subconsciously believed that it was difficult to raise her leg, nor that as a result of this belief she was putting far too much effort into a simple motion. When she realized how difficult it was to even imagine lifting her leg, her whole attitude changed. She realized immediately how much her mind affected her body's movement.

Once someone recognizes her problems and their causes, it is much easier to find a solution. The therapist's main job is to help the patient increase her awareness. Visualization is an effective tool for this. I have found it to be most effective when used in conjunction with massage and movement. If a patient has tense leg muscles, the therapist may hold and gently stretch the leg while asking the patient to imagine that the muscles are growing longer, lighter, and looser, or that the breath is flowing into the tight muscles, through the leg, and out of the feet. In nearly every case, the muscles will indeed lengthen and relax.

The therapist must, of course, be creative. No single visualization exercise is right for every patient, and it is up to the therapist to determine which imagery will help the patient. Once she learned how helpful visualization was, Naomi continued to use it along with her exercises with great success, until gradually her back became strong and healthy.

Increasing Your Awareness of Your Body

BEFORE MOVING to the United States, I thought that I could only educate people individually, since in my sessions I always tailored the movement exercises to my clients' individual needs. But my clients and students in the United States asked me to teach classes. I was reluctant at first, until I realized that even people with different needs and problems have a lot in common. One important thing almost everyone has in common is a lack of familiarity with their bodies. Building up people's awareness — making the connection between the mind and the body — was necessary. It was also possible to do it in a class situation, no less so than in individual sessions.

Before you can visualize your movement getting better, you need to learn how your body conducts itself in the first place. When you better understand how your body organizes its functioning, you become aware of what you are doing in a harmful way, what you are doing in a useful fashion, and where you can use imagery to change. I believe that a lack of such consciousness causes many of the modern ailments, from back problems to spine injuries, from visual stress to loss of vision, from poor circulation to heart disease, from stiffness to arthritis.

In one of my classes, a woman whose legs were paralyzed complained that her paralysis had extended into her arms. During the course of the class, we found that the stiffness in her back caused the limitation of movement in her arms. When she increased the mobility in her back, her arms moved normally. In a way, this is what happens to all of us. We use only certain parts of our bodies, putting tremendous stress on those parts, and we need to learn to move the parts that we tend to neglect.

Relearning to Walk

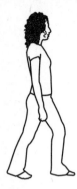

ONE OF MY FAVORITE exercises to teach in workshops is relearning to walk. It is important to learn how to walk better, since a stiff gait can hurt the feet, the knees, the hip joints, and the back. The foot needs to be fully mobile, as the weight in walking is transferred from the heel to the toes. The knee should be bent when it is in front of you, and straightened when it is behind you. But when you observe people walking, you can read in their posture so much about their self-esteem, social status or affiliation, day-to-day worries, and self-consciousness. Try to correct a stiff gait, and you face all these elements as hurdles in your way. You can spend all day doing that with minimal results.

On the other hand, none of us has any such limiting dictates when it comes to walking backward. So when I take a group of people out to the park or the beach, we walk or run backward. This is an opportunity to explore groups of muscles — the back of the legs, the gluteals, the back — and bring them to the attention of the brain. We walk backward, stop, feel the back, pay attention to the posture being straighter, walk backward again, notice that the leg we land on is bent, and then try to walk forward. Walking forward is very different at this point; the brain finds it easier to employ the leg joints fully. At this point, one is more likely to step forward with a bent knee, rather than a stiff one.

Another reason this exercise is effective for many people is that when we walk forward, we pay attention to what we see ahead of us. Our bodies may have the habit of contracting themselves as part of the way we use our eyes. Walking backward, we peek once in a while, but most of the time our eyes are relaxed, joining us for the ride like passengers; we let go of the tension associated with using our eyes.

Working with Underused Muscles

ROLLING FROM SIDE TO SIDE is another important exercise that I've used in my classes; it helps the participants familiarize themselves with another group of muscles they're normally not aware of. The following is a variation of the exercise called "Rolling from Side to Side" that I described in chapter 9 (Back Problems).

Body Awareness Exercise: Rolling from Side to Side

Find a quiet space, lie on your back on a mat or a carpet, and massage your abdomen. Now roll from side to side: Roll to the right until your left hand touches the floor in front of your chest, then push yourself away to start rolling to the left. Now push yourself with your right hand to start your roll to the right. Also let your hips and legs gently push you from side to side. Pay attention to the sides of your body as you roll. Because so much of our normal movement is forward, rolling from side to side may feel odd.

Now lie on one side, stretch your arms above your head, interlace your fingers, and roll for a moment, just a little, back and forth, on the ribs of that side. Turn onto your other side, again stretch your arms above your head with your fingers interlaced, and resume rolling from side to side. You may find that rolling is easier now.

We tend to limit the neural pathways that we use in our movement. When we perform an exercise such as rolling from side to side, we activate muscles that we have neglected, and we create new neural pathways for them. When, in addition, we let go of unnecessary muscle contraction in our bodies, we integrate those newly activated muscles into our day-to-day movement.

To a great extent, function leads to structure. Most people you see are stooped forward. They weren't born that way. Most people suffer from back pain. That's not because we're born to have back pain; it's because of poor use of the body. We tend to overuse some of our muscles and underuse others. Some of our muscles remain overly contracted, while others become weak. The patterns of movement that lead to this imbalance become more rigid with time. They reinforce the problems that develop in the body. But these patterns can be changed through functioning differently. This new functioning comes from breaking existing patterns and putting a tremendous amount of thought and care into creating new ways of coordinating our movements. When we function differently, all the back pain and tension we may have carried for years can surely leave our bodies.

You cannot move your body mechanically, without awareness of it, and expect not to cause yourself damage. On the other hand, the combination of imagination and awareness will help you maintain and increase your body's health. It is wrong to overcontract the muscles, and it is wrong to overstretch them. If you overcontract your muscles, you may not be able to stretch them. If you overstretch your muscles, you may not be able to contract them. It is also wrong to move the body in a limited way that repeats itself all the time. For example, most of us are overflexing. We write, drive, walk, wash dishes, and sit while bending forward, even if slightly. To compensate for that, we need to stretch backward and to the sides; we need to find the muscles we neglect and use them.

Here are a few more body-awareness exercises that I've used in many of my classes.

Body Awareness Exercise: Centering and Expanding

This is an important exercise. Sit on a comfortable chair and imagine that your head goes up to the sky. Imagine that one shoulder stretches as far as one side of the room, while the other shoulder reaches the other side of the room. Visualize your back lengthening and the spaces between your vertebrae increasing. Breathe deeply and slowly, in and out through your nose. Inhale slowly, and exhale even more slowly.

At the same time, imagine that there is a direct connection between the center of your body (the area of your navel) and the center of the earth. If you can imagine such a connection but you don't really feel it, that's a good start, but it may not create a huge change in your body. You can achieve a sense of centering only when your joints are loose; your neck feels expansive, your vertebrae feel separated from each other; your shoulders feel far apart from each other; there is more space in your pelvis; your legs, thighs, and feet feel elongated; and your whole body feels wide and long. This feeling of expansion is what leads to centering. Similarly, it's impossible to maintain the sense of expansion without feeling centered. Therefore, we need to work on both of these elements together: the expansion and the centering. The attempt to become centered and expansive can help you feel which tensions stand in your way and which movements you need to make.

So sit and imagine that your head goes up, one shoulder extends in one direction, the other shoulder extends in the other direction, and there is a large space between one vertebra and another.

Keep that thought with you all the time. When you walk, imagine that your head goes up to the sky, one shoulder stretches to one side of the universe, and the other shoulder stretches to the other side of the universe. We do have a technical problem, in that gravity pulls us down but the sky doesn't lift us up to balance that pull. Many forms of bodywork strive to achieve that lifting balance by using the same thought: Stretch yourself up with the help of your imagination. This helps us counteract not just gravity, but the other forces that pull us down and make us feel small, stooped, and cramped — namely, life's troubles. If you remember to expand toward the sky and toward both sides of the universe just a few times a day, you'll create more separation between your vertebrae, your brain will allow your movement to be more fluid and light, and you will feel a huge difference in your ability to function well.

Body Awareness Exercise: Separating Leg and Back Functions

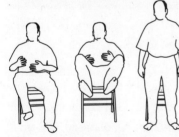

Now sit on a chair, tap on your abdomen, and, at the same time, tap the bottoms of your feet on the floor one by one for about a minute. This will call your attention to your center and your feet. Now lift both your legs up together and stand up at once, hitting the floor with both feet. You may notice that the act of standing up did not involve effort from your back, as it otherwise would have. Because you paid attention to your feet, you created more of a separation between the function of your legs and the function of your back, and you didn't unnecessarily recruit back muscles that weren't needed for the act of standing. Walk around the room now, paying attention to placing your foot heel first, then bringing your weight toward your toes. Have a sense of lightness and ease in your gait.

Here's another way to create a separation between the function of the legs and that of the back: Stand and tap your feet against the floor.

Then, when you walk, imagine that your feet are lifting your legs. For example, when I run on San Francisco's sandy beaches, I imagine that the sand is like a trampoline, bouncing my legs up after every step I make. Of course, the feet cannot actually be carrying the legs along. But when you imagine that they do, you let go of many of the muscles you've been tensing in your back and your abdomen as you walk. This way, you allow the ankle muscles, knees, and hip joints to work independently from the lower, middle, and upper back and the neck. This is such a relief for the back!

Body Awareness Exercise: Forearm Rotation

Lie on your back with a small pillow under your head. Rest your elbows at your sides, on the floor or mat. As a starting position, rest both hands on your diaphragm. Now start to rotate your forearms in large circles, with your elbows remaining on the floor or mat. Rotate the arms about twenty-five times in each direction.

Now add another movement to the rotation: Roll your head from side to side. Try to let go of your head and not tense your neck. Don't press your head heavily on the pillow or try to wring your neck. This time, as you rotate your forearms imagine that your fingertips are carrying your arms along, rather than muscles in your arms or shoulders. We're taking imagery a step farther in these exercises, and combining it with movement. You may want to think of yourself as a marionette, with your fingertips attached to strings. Although the movement remains the same, allowing yourself to let go of the muscles in your shoulders and arms — even if only in your mind — will actually make a difference in your muscle recruitment. Your shoulders will let go of a lot of stress.

Stop the movement for a little while; just imagine that your forearms are continuing to move, that your head rolls easily from side to side, and that the movement is easy and smooth. Now continue to actually rotate your forearms, and you will probably find that your forearms feel lighter and your neck feels looser as you move your head from side to side.

The last step of this exercise adds another element. While moving your head and forearms as before, concentrate on your back. Imagine that your back is being stretched, becoming both longer and wider.

While some people find it easy to visualize a movement, others find it practically impossible. If you can't visualize a movement you wish to perform, vocalize what you are trying to imagine. Say out loud, "I am rotating my forearms," and you may find that when you do the actual movement again, it will be easier. This technique has worked for thousands of people in my classes, just like it worked many years ago for Mr. Shadmi.

Body Awareness Exercise: Leg Rotation

Lie on your front and concentrate on your legs, all the way from your hip joints to your knees, and from your knees to your feet. Now bend one knee and rotate your calf in both directions, with your foot drawing a large circle in the air. Imagine that the foot is leading the motion; breathe deeply and slowly. Now stop and rest your leg, either by keeping it bent or by bringing your foot back down to the mat. Imagine that you are rotating your calf again, in both directions.

Take a rest from this visualization and pay attention to your leg. Does it feel longer? When we stand and walk, our legs are so often straight — in knee extension — that they feel wonderful when we give them a break from the effort and tightness involved.

Now imagine again that you are rotating your calf, as before, in both directions. Now stop the visualization and actually rotate your foot at the ankle, in both directions. Imagine that your foot is leading the motion and that you don't need to use the muscles of your calf and shin for the motion.

Now rotate your calf at the knee; your leg may feel even longer than before. Rotate it six to eight times in each direction, and imagine that your foot is leading the motion. Bring your leg down to the floor or mat, and notice whether it feels longer than the leg you haven't exercised yet.

Repeat the entire exercise with your other leg. When you're done, bend both knees and rotate your calves together in both directions,

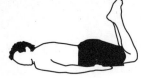

imagining that your feet are leading the motion. Now bring both legs down, and notice whether your legs feel longer and stretched.

We tend to be unaware of how much motion is indeed available to our bodies. The following two exercises can demonstrate that.

Body Awareness Exercise: Stretching Your Arms Back

Stand and open your arms wide, with your palms facing forward. Try to stretch your arms back, at shoulder level. How far can they go? Have you reached your limit? Now turn your head toward one stretched arm, and imagine it going just a little farther. Can you indeed stretch it just a little more? Turn your head to the other side and look at your other arm. Can you imagine it going just a little farther back? Try to move it beyond where it is now. Return to the first arm you looked at, and try this again. After several such attempts, you may find that your arms are stretched far beyond the place you originally defined as your limit. Now let your arms relax.

Body Awareness Exercise: Swinging Your Legs

Stand on your right foot and swing your left leg from left to right, and right to left, about thirty times. When you swing your leg to the right, swing it in front of your body. You will need to bend your left knee a little to do that. As your leg swings away from your body, you are using your abductor muscles. As your leg swings in front of you, you are using your adductors. This both helps loosen your hip joint and strengthen those side muscles of the leg, which are important for stabilizing your leg.

Now swing your leg forward and back about thirty times. This creates flexion and extension of the hip joint. You want to have a sense of the full motion available to your hip joint.

Once in a while, as you do both swings, tap your left foot on the floor several times. This will help you visualize that the foot is leading the motion.

Repeat the whole process, standing on your left foot and swinging your right leg.

Now walk, paying attention to the muscles you are using to support your walk. You will have an easier time lifting your foot now, since you've reminded the brain to recruit your abductors and adductors to do the work as well. You've also allowed the brain to let go of the back muscles it may have unnecessarily involved in the process of walking.

When we use the local leg muscles as much as possible, we are less likely to recruit the back muscles to support leg movement. As we separate and isolate muscle groups, we better control the muscles we use, and we let go of the muscles we don't really need for the particular motion. Visualizing such isolation is an important tool in making the movement smoother; it helps achieve a sense of elongation, and it relieves overcontraction of the back. This isolation prevents the joints from tightening and jamming, and is therefore an important element in the prevention of arthritis and spine problems. Isolation also better activates the nervous system, as it brings about more variability of movement. For people with vulnerable nervous systems, this can mean the difference between maintaining their health and developing neurological disorders, such as multiple sclerosis. If you already have arthritis, back problems, or neurological problems, the isolation of your muscles can be very useful in your recovery process.

Body Awareness Exercise: Isolating Parts of the Back

This exercise will help you isolate and move separate parts of your back. Get on your hands and knees and move your lower back up and down. It may be hard to separate your lower 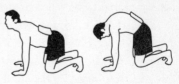 back from the rest of your back in your mind. In that case, place a large book or a long, narrow sandbag on your lower back; now move the lower back up and down, with the weight helping you sense where your lower back is actually located.

Do the same thing with the middle of your back, then with your upper back — the area between your shoulders.

Release of Stored Emotions

IT IS AMAZING how emotionally invested we are in not moving many parts of our bodies. In a 1982 workshop I gave in Fresno, California, I demonstrated an exercise to mobilize the chest: We stood facing the wall, placed our palms against the wall, and moved our chests back and forth. The chest is an area where we tend to lock up strong emotions. We touched our chests and the middle of our backs with our thumbs to give us a tactile sense of the chest movement we were practicing. We then tapped our fingertips against our thighs or against the wall, just to have a sense of our fingertips, then rotated our arms in large circles, imagining that our fingertips were leading the motion. After loosening our shoulders in this fashion, we returned to moving our chests back and forth.

One of the participants — a very sweet woman — started crying at this point. But that didn't prepare us for what happened when we moved on to an exercise that isolated the toes. We were moving our toes one at a time by holding onto four of them and rotating only one. We pressed on each toe in different directions, trying to move the toe up, down, left, and right against resistance.

When we stood up, the same woman who had cried earlier became pale, then collapsed on the couch. In her delirium, she cried out, "Stop the fire!" She seemed unconscious of her surroundings — only of her inner reality. Several people tried to tell her that there was no fire, but she didn't seem to hear. I asked one of the participants to quickly bring me a jug of water. When the water arrived, we poured it on her toes. She appeared to be relieved, and she slowly came to.

She seemed calm, and was surprised to see everyone standing around looking at her. She had no idea what had happened. When we told her about it, she said, "I can't believe it. A year ago my house was on fire, and my toes were burned and painful. I appeared to be strong, and I took care of everything, but apparently I carried with me this incredible fear that my toes were going to get burned." Her toes had mostly healed from the burns, but they weren't completely recovered at the time of the workshop. But the fear hadn't gone away as easily as the burns had healed. The exercise that released the chest had allowed emotions trapped there to surface.

Powerful emotions that you experienced in the past may have shaped your posture then. Your fear, grief, anger, or hurt locked themselves into your muscles by contracting them. They may have caused narrowing of the chest, rounding of the shoulders, or tightening of the abdomen, buttocks, thighs, jaw, neck, face, forehead, or scalp. They may have led to constant fidgeting, doodling, wriggling of the toes, or squeezing of the face with every blink. These postural adaptations and automatic movements, which you may not even be aware of, can remain with you for years after the events that caused them are no longer relevant to your life.

Current events in your life can trigger emotions of a great magnitude. These emotions may, in some cases, be unrelated to your present; you may have carried them for years in your muscles. Do you ever find yourself responding with anger, fear, or sadness, out of proportion to a particular problem you are facing? Movement that releases the tension in your muscles may trigger the old emotions locked in them, bringing the feelings to the surface. With more movement, those feelings can evaporate — just go away. It may not be an easy process to go through, but it is a very important one.

When you work on increasing movement in your body, it can be very effective in releasing your emotions. I therefore suggest that, in times of emotional change, you talk to a spiritual guide, a psychotherapist, or a good friend, and that you keep a journal to record your emotional changes and your awareness.

The Role of Imagery

IN MY TEACHING, I have incorporated imagery into most exercises. With almost every exercise you do, you can imagine doing things differently than you're accustomed to. In general, you may want to imagine that the movement you are performing is not done with the central, large, over-recruited muscles. The image of the marionette that I introduced earlier can be used in many other forms of movement.

Body Awareness Exercise: Easier Imagery

For example, lie on your back with your knees bent and move your legs together from side to side, bringing your knees toward the floor on either side. Difficult? It doesn't have to be. Now imagine that your knees are leading the motion, your legs are lifting themselves, and the muscles of your abdomen are not necessary for the movement at all.

To make this even easier, you need to make the visualization easier. So tap your knees against each other a few times in order to have a sensation in your knees, and therefore a better connection between your knees and your mind. Now move your knees from side to side again while your abdomen rests.

I encourage you to create new exercises and the imagery that goes with them. There is another important thing to remember when you do that: Don't attempt what you cannot achieve. Don't visualize something that is beyond your reach. Take the next step. If you try to visualize something that is beyond your reach, your subconscious will immediately reject your conscious visualization. If you visualize a slight improvement, you won't trigger subconscious rejection; your visualization will be effective, and you will see improvement. When you try to accomplish everything at once, you're in fact challenging the process; if you take it a step at a time, you are able to trust that the process will work.

Not only does function lead to structure, but thought leads to new ways of functioning. In the brain, for every two neurons that receive information from our senses, we have five motor neurons that instruct the muscles to contract and 200,000 interneurons. The interneurons receive information from the sensory neurons and communicate with one another until they form an order to send to the motor neurons. Most of our movement is not automatic; it results from thinking, sensing, and patterns that we've developed and learned. Our thoughts and imagery can change the movement commands that our brain sends to our body. I've seen other methods of bodywork and movement therapy that concentrate on breaking movement patterns, but some of them don't offer suggestions for healthy, effective patterns to incorporate in their place. We want to develop patterns that lead to more mobility, more flexibility, and greater awareness.

Imagery can be effective, not just for improving movement, but for improving eyesight, breathing, and circulation. We need to remember that, just as we can visualize ourselves moving better and feeling better, we need to give up on our old images and expectations of limited movement, pain, and deterioration. These images may be imposed on us by other people's thoughts, especially as we advance in age. These negative images are often in our way, and we need to familiarize ourselves with them in order to learn how to let them go.

In summary, we can use visualization of a specific movement that we are about to perform in order to help us do it more easily or smoothly. We can also visualize a movement before performing it, in order to sense in advance where we may tense ourselves or where our movement may lack grace; we can then perform the actual movement with more fluidity. Visualization can also be used while moving to make the movement easier, lighter, and more efficient. The ability to visualize can be learned. Some people have an easier time than others, but everyone I've met has been able to improve his or her skills.

CHAPTER 13

MUSCULAR DYSTROPHY

The Vegetarian Society hosted many conferences on health and medicine, attended by prestigious physicians and health-care professionals. It was at one of these conferences that Danny, Vered, and I originally met Dr. Arkin, the neurologist, who also practiced acupuncture.

Although Vered's improvement was remarkable, she still limped heavily. Vered and I told Dr. Arkin what we had done for her so far, and asked him if he could do anything for her leg. He was interested, and he invited the three of us to his home to meet with him informally.

Dr. Arkin examined my eyes and was stunned when he saw the fragmented lenses. "With these lenses, you should be completely blind," he told me.

When he examined Vered, Dr. Arkin told us that acupuncture couldn't increase Vered's mobility, and that our method was probably the best thing in the world for her.

However, Dr. Arkin was particularly interested in Danny. In Danny's pilgrimage from clinic to clinic in search of a cure, he had been to Dr. Arkin's clinic. As a result, Dr. Arkin had access to Danny's records. Dr. Arkin was impressed by the muscle development in his arms and thighs. He could see at once that Danny had built up muscles that were underdeveloped in most people, to substitute for muscles that had deteriorated. More than anything else, the enormous improvements Danny had made convinced Dr. Arkin of the value of our work.

The Nature of Muscular Dystrophy

DANNY HAD BEEN DIAGNOSED with Duchenne muscular dystrophy. Muscular dystrophy is a group of genetic diseases with one thing in common: These patients have fragile muscles, easily damaged by the activities of daily life. In Duchenne, as well as many of the other forms of muscular dystrophy, the normal attachment of a tough, protective outer layer to the muscle is absent. In people who don't have muscular dystrophy, this protein-chain attachment pins the protective layer to the muscle fiber, penetrating the soft outer membrane of the muscle fiber and clamping onto the cell's internal architecture. Different links of the chain are missing in each form of muscular dystrophy, but the result is pretty much the same. The protein may also be present but defective; this makes a huge difference in the course of the disease.

This protective layer is a life-or-death matter to the muscle fiber, because muscles work by deforming (changing shape) while developing force, often against considerable resistance. For the healthy person, muscles get bigger and stronger when we work them hard, but for the muscular dystrophy patient, all but the gentlest movements are destructive.

Severity and life expectancy differ enormously among the different forms of muscular dystrophy. Some babies die of muscular dystrophy in the womb or are never able to leave the hospital where they are born. The later symptoms appear in a person's life, the more promising the outcome. Some of these diseases, such as fascioscapulohumeral (FSHD) muscular dystrophy, have extremely varied manifestations; the parent may have lost only the ability to whistle, while the child struggles to eat, walk, reach objects on shelves, or lift things.

Duchenne muscular dystrophy is the most common neuromuscular disease of childhood. Caused by a defect in the X chromosome, it is carried by the mother and manifests as disease in the son. About one-third of these boys suffer from mental retardation, and many have cardiac problems. Invariably, symptoms like clumsiness and frequent falls appear at around age three; if the disease has not previously appeared in the family, this is often the first time they are aware of a problem. The boy is then usually in a wheelchair by the age of ten or twelve, and death generally occurs by his early twenties. The cause of death is almost always either a heart problem or pneumonia; if the breathing muscles aren't strong enough to produce a good cough, pathogens from the throat can migrate into the lungs, and antibiotics are ineffective against some of these microbes.

Even though a lot of brilliant research has been performed, the medical profession still has no cure for any form of muscular dystrophy. Doctors are forced to tell parents of youngsters who have Duchenne and closely related forms of muscular dystrophy that there is no hope — that they can expect to see progressive losses, and eventually death.

Mr. Kominski: Function Restored

DR. ARKIN REFERRED a patient to us who had an unusual case of muscular dystrophy. Mr. Kominski was fifty years old when he came to us. The process of deterioration had begun when he was twenty, and developed slowly over thirty years. Until a year earlier, he had seemed almost normal, but then his condition worsened dramatically. Mr. Kominski owned a small citrus farm, and he began to have difficulty picking fruit because he could barely lift his arms. He had consulted several doctors, and even faith healers, to no avail.

I tested Mr. Kominski's muscles and found that his pectoral muscles were very contracted and had almost completely atrophied. His throat was so tight that he could hardly speak. His arm muscles, too, were tight and hard, and he could barely move his arms. The few leg muscles he could still use were extremely tight, even when he was at rest; this indicated that they were working far beyond their capacity.

I told Mr. Kominski that he had to stop pushing himself beyond his limits when his muscles were in such a state of exhaustion. Our first suggestion was that he immediately stop certain activities, particularly the hard labor of caring for his orchard and fields. He needed to become aware of his weakness and then work on strengthening himself.

I went to work massaging Mr. Kominski's muscles; this was a great relief to him, but it took several sessions before the results of the treatment showed. Gradually, he began to function better and feel more energetic. We grew to like each other very much.

At our suggestion, Mr. Kominski consulted Dr. Frumer for advice about a natural diet. He began a diet of simple, unprocessed foods; this helped his worn-out body by making digestion easier and lowering the level of toxic material his body had to eliminate. Mr. Kominski's main problem was that he simply had no idea what was helpful for his body and what was not.

After only three weeks, Mr. Kominski had improved significantly; he found it much easier to use his arms, to walk, and to function in general. He went to his neurologist, Dr. Kotter, to show her how much he'd improved. As the chief neurologist at her hospital, she had a staff of thirteen neurologists working under her. She called a meeting to show them, along with a group of medical students, the improvement in Mr. Kominski's muscles. His case seemed to confirm her own thinking: that what a patient with muscular dystrophy needs most of all is the right kind of movement therapy.

Dr. Kotter asked to meet us. This made me nervous, as I was barely twenty and completely without conventional training. I called Dr. Arkin, and he reassured me that Dr. Kotter was a very open-minded person, and that I should by all means meet with her.

Our visit with Dr. Kotter was cordial. The first thing we did was to show her Danny's medical history; she was so impressed with his progress that she expressed doubts that he'd ever had muscular dystrophy. Given that she was the chief neurologist of a major hospital, she gave us quite a compliment when she said, "One thing I know for sure: You three are authentic. There is a lot that you don't know, and I will straighten you out anytime you say something that doesn't make sense to me as a doctor. But I like what you are doing, and I will refer patients to you to see what sort of results you get."

Lili: From Near Paralysis to Walking

A FEW WEEKS LATER, Dr. Kotter referred Lili to us. She told Lili's father that nothing medical could be done to help his daughter, who suffered from muscular dystrophy. "As for nutrition, you can feed her any soup you want, but I don't think it will help either. But I do know three young people who might be able to help her. If you see them, please tell me the results."

Lili was five years old. She had shown the first symptoms of muscular dystrophy at eighteen months, and had already outlived her first doctor's prognosis. Although she could barely crawl, her parents never got her a wheelchair, suspecting that this might cause her psychological trauma. I was pleased about this, because sitting in a wheelchair would have robbed her of what little opportunity she had for movement.

Lili was very weak, and her body was thin and deformed. Her hands flopped at her sides and could not be held forward. Her shoulder blades and collarbone bulged out, barely covered with skin. Her lower back was curved backward, while her upper back was curved forward. Her neck was so weak that her head lolled forward on her chest. When she crawled, it was with an ineffective sideways groping, rather than straight forward like a normal child. She was barely breathing.

The first time we tested Lili, we found that it was difficult for her to lift her arms. She couldn't move them at all against any resistance. She also couldn't lift her legs, and when we asked her to lie on her stomach and bend her knee, she could only raise the foot a few inches. Any normal motion was nearly impossible for her. She had no strength in her body.

We decided to use massage and passive movement — movement performed by the therapist rather than the patient, with the therapist holding part of the patient's body and gently moving it. This is different from physical therapy, in which the patient is usually encouraged to strenuously work a weak muscle. We tried to move Lili's weak muscles in the easiest way possible, then show her how to continue this movement on her own.

We showed her mother how to rotate Lili's foot, then her leg, knee, elbow, and arm, then each toe and finger, while Lili lay on her back moving her head from side to side. After two sessions, Lili's mother called to tell us that Lili had remembered all the exercises; she'd even corrected some errors her mother had made in helping her. Lili was wonderfully alert and perceptive; after a couple of sessions, she became enthusiastic about her treatment and her exercises. I would say that she sensed a great change coming, and this awareness helped end her process of decay.

After three sessions, Lili suffered no further loss of function. With her mother's help, she did four hours of exercise each day. By the end of our fifth session, she could lie on her back and lift her leg to a right angle with her body, and she could lift her arms straight above her head. Her neck muscles also began to gain in strength and mobility, although her head still drooped forward. After seven sessions, she could crawl on her hands and knees like a normal child.

A few weeks after our first session, Lili took her first steps in three years. She still had a pronounced swayback, which made it difficult for her to stand up, so I supported her back. I had one hand on her back and my other hand on her abdomen — and she took a few steps!

Less than a week later, Lili was able, with some support, to walk down the stairs to her mother's car. This was the most rapid, dramatic progress I had ever seen with a muscular dystrophy patient. The joy of seeing this little girl on her feet was so powerful that it has never left me. She was one of our most astonishing cases. It took only twenty-one days for her transformation from near paralysis to walking.

Needless to say, our work with Lili won us the respect of Dr. Kotter, who began to refer more patients to us. It was a pleasure to work in harmony with the established medical community. We wanted to reach as many people as possible, and the support of physicians was very helpful.

Our Approach to Muscular Dystrophy

THE SELF-HEALING program for muscular dystrophy combines massage, breathing, movement exercises, and lifestyle changes.

It is important to carefully evaluate the muscles of a muscular dystrophy patient to find out which ones are healthy, which are healthy but tight, and which are dystrophic, or damaged. The muscles damaged by the disease may either be atrophied (thin and wasted) or pseudohypertrophic, which means that they are enlarged but weak. Pseudohypertrophic muscles may look strong and well shaped, like well-developed muscles, but in fact they are weak because much of the muscle tissue has been replaced by fat and connective tissue. I am more concerned about pseudohypertrophic muscles than about the atrophied ones, because in such cases the muscle fibers that are still functional are burdened with the weight of the fat and connective tissue that surround them.

The stronger muscles of a muscular dystrophy patient, which compensate for the muscles ravaged by the disease, may already be suffering from the disease to some extent, or they may be the next to be attacked. In order to improve circulation for both the strong muscles and the dystrophic muscles adjacent to them, we begin treatment by relieving tension and stiffness in these strong, tense muscles with massage, passive movement, and stretches.

Self-Healing massage for dystrophic muscles is always very light. We use several techniques that help the muscles "puff up" as their tone improves. It takes a lot of massage to support muscular dystrophy patients, so I always try to recruit their families and friends to join my sessions and continue the work at home.

The sensitivity of the massage therapist's touch is critical. Some muscles will require the gentlest touch, others a firmer pressure. Massage can both relax dystrophic muscle and strengthen it. But a touch that is rough and insensitive can damage dystrophic muscle. In fact, even the gentlest touch to a muscle that is not ready for it can be damaging.

When the client is strong enough, I introduce passive movement into the session. The client needs to let go of a limb and become like a rag doll while the limb is moved, usually in a circular motion. Many people find it a considerable challenge to completely relax a limb and trust someone else to move it. When clients do relax, they discover that passive movement reaccustoms their muscles to movement without requiring them to struggle against gravity or resistance, and therefore without fatiguing them. Stretches are part of this phase of therapy; they increase flexibility and range of movement at the joints.

Active movement often begins with water exercises, in warm pools or bathtubs. We find movements that are easy and begin with few repetitions, then build up the number of repetitions as endurance increases over time, up to hundreds. Water exercises are extremely relaxing and rejuvenating.

People with muscular dystrophy need to avoid hard manual labor and generally guard against overuse, repetitive strain, and immobility. Above all, they need to always stay below their fatigue level. Exercises for muscular dystrophy patients must be individualized in order to avoid causing harm, so I am not providing any here.

Rosie: From Canes to Dancing

ROSIE WAS NEVER GOOD at sports in school. In fact, people always told her she was slow and lazy. In her late teens, she was diagnosed with FSHD.

When I first met Rosie, she was thirty-three years old. She walked with much difficulty, using two canes to support herself. She fell frequently. As a schoolteacher, she had her students write essays about "whacky the cane" or "my teacher has wobbly legs."

Rosie met me at a workshop I was teaching in London, then traveled to Tel Aviv to work with me there as a guest of my advanced training class. She later came to work with me in San Francisco several times, and worked regularly with my students and graduates in London.

After coming to see me, Rosie took up a daily program of movement exercises, mostly in a warm pool, where she gradually built up her repetitions of gentle, circular motions. She spent about two hours a day at the pool; it eventually became an important part of her social life, and the members of the swim club even raised funds for one of her San Francisco trips.

I made a point of traveling to England for Rosie's fortieth birthday, where she was able to demonstrate to her many friends that she could even dance! Over ten years, Rosie was able to improve her walking dramatically. At that point, her condition leveled off, and her gait deteriorated to some extent. Rosie took it upon herself to help spread the word about the Self-Healing Method. She told people about it, became a research subject, and made her home in London available for the practice of Self-Healing.

Beatriz: Amazing the Specialists

IN 1988, I was invited to Brazil to spend a week working with muscular dystrophy patients. One of the people I worked with was Beatriz Nascimento, a bright young assistant professor of occupational therapy. Like Rosie, she suffered from FSHD. I saw Beatriz in Brazil for a few sessions. She was very concerned about her disease because her mother, who had the same disease, was close to needing a wheelchair. FSHD typically shows up as deterioration of the facial muscles, upper arms, and upper back. Like Rosie, Beatriz was suffering from muscle loss in her legs as well.

Beatriz had lost several functions and found herself becoming increasingly limited: She used to dance samba, but she couldn't do that anymore. She used to participate in political groups, but now even raising her arm was no longer possible. Chewing became difficult, so even the pleasure of eating was gone. She had lost over twenty pounds just because her chewing muscles had become too weak to function.

After my first few sessions in São Paulo, Beatriz was still sad, but hopeful; her legs started feeling much better very quickly. She decided to come to San Francisco for more therapy and for training. Within a few months, she overcame the bureaucratic hurdles and arrived in San Francisco to research my work, sponsored by the Federal University of São Carlos.

In her sessions, I discovered that passive movement was very effective for Beatriz. I worked on her weak deltoid muscles, and I had her lift her arm while lying on her back, which was easier than while standing. I relaxed her weak shins by shaking them. She also needed a lot of facial massage. She not only had difficulty eating, but she complained that she couldn't smile; the sides of her mouth couldn't come up because of the weakness of her cheeks.

For six months, Beatriz spent two and a half hours a day working on herself. By the end of that period, she could lift her arms almost normally, eat all she wanted, dance again, and smile a lot. She became a teacher of the Self-Healing Method, and regularly offers Self-Healing training to students of occupational and physical therapy at the University of São Carlos. She also cofounded a free clinic for muscular dystrophy at the university.

Thirteen years after Beatriz first started working with this method, specialists in Brazil were amazed by her test results, compared to their notes from 1989. She had regained almost all the function that she had lost by 1989, and maintained her improvements for thirteen years, while slowly getting stronger. Without therapy, she was expected to deteriorate at about 4 percent per year.

CHAPTER 14

SUCCESSFUL AGING

Many years ago, my friend Arnon said to me, "I can no longer run like I used to when I was eighteen. My body's getting old." He was twenty-four.

Was he really getting old? Perhaps he was a little stiffer than he'd been at eighteen, and he might have injured himself through physical activities in the intervening years. But the main thing that stopped him from running as well as he did at eighteen was his expectation that he would deteriorate with time.

This chapter is for those of you who are hoping to prepare yourselves for aging well, as well as for anyone who is supporting an older relative or friend in their aging process.

It is true that our bodies change over time. We don't mount as strong a response to physiological challenges in our later years as we do in our youth. Our genes dictate that we will age and eventually die. But most people die too young. At any time, you can work on improving the quality of your life and increasing your chances of living longer. Your potential for improvement may be limited, or it may be beyond your expectation; either way, it is never too late — or too early — to get started.

In your twenties or thirties, you might have the feeling that you can get away with eating junk food, smoking, or not exercising; you might still feel fine and go about your activities without difficulty. You may have gotten away with it, or you may just have imagined that you did, while developing atherosclerosis or the beginning of another chronic illness. But in either case, you can't get away with it forever. By the time you're in your forties or fifties, you'll realize that your body is no longer so forgiving.

Overcoming Destructive Habits

TOO OFTEN, I hear people say that they know they're harming themselves with one bad habit or another, but they just can't — really can't — quit. And then I meet people who do quit smoking, drinking alcohol, or eating junk food — sometimes overnight after they got scared enough, such as after their first stroke or heart attack. To my great pleasure, I also meet people who decide to change their lifestyle without the threat of scary symptoms.

My work is mainly in the field of movement and exercise, but I have to bring up the issues of smoking and diet. There isn't anyone who really can't quit a bad habit, even if their list of excuses is long. It is our human will, deep in our minds — perhaps even our soul — that makes it possible to change our lives. Even if you've been drinking coffee for fifty or eighty years, today is the day to stop. Even if you've smoked since you were a preteen, or have been eating fried food all your life, now is the time to change that. When you take such a step, you may suffer a little, but you will achieve a lot. For one thing, if your poor dietary habits cause discomfort such as fatigue, indigestion, or excess weight, a better diet will give you a sense of well-being that will make it easier for you to follow an exercise program. On top of that, you will appreciate yourself and increase your self-esteem for having shown control, and you will feel much more capable of carrying on with your life's goals and tasks.

If you have poor or destructive habits that you would like to change, don't take them on all at once. Decide on your next step and take it today. One goal at a time will do.

There is a big difference between enjoying a slice of birthday cake on occasion and needing a sugar or chocolate fix daily. And it is hard to do something you've been addicted to in moderation. I recommend staying away from things you find difficult to avoid — for months or even a couple of years — before allowing yourself to have some on occasion.

How do you know if something you're consuming is harmful to you? Educate yourself. But more than that, ask yourself if what you're consuming causes you fatigue, irritability, heartburn, or poor sleep. Our bodies are not all the same, and dietary needs vary from one person to another. I won't go into specific suggestions here, other than to mention a few items that, in my opinion, should be on the top of your list of things to avoid: fried foods, excess sugar and salt, and anything addictive, such as alcohol, coffee, or chocolate.

The transition is difficult, but it's rewarding.

Mobility

THERE ARE SEVERAL other elements of aging well. I'd like to start with one of my favorite subjects: mobility. Many of the people I meet do not pay attention to the creeping stiffness in their bodies. While smoking cigarettes and drinking coffee can lead to stiffness, and poor movement habits can lead to arthritis, the most important element is one's attitude. Even young people often accept stiffness as a fact of life. If you don't pay attention to your body's stiffening, you'll develop arthritis. If you pay attention but have all the excuses about why you won't do something about it, you'll develop arthritis just the same. In my opinion, stiffness will determine what your aging process will be like even more than the foods you eat.

Assuming that you want to live a long life while feeling as young as possible, you need to be responsible about the route you take — and it's good to start early. It takes more than good genes and luck to do well later in life; research has shown that social support, hope, and reduced stress are important elements in aging well.

What does all that have to do with stiffness? Everything. The more mobility one has, the more one is likely to go out and socialize. The greater one's mobility, the better one's circulation, including, of course, the health of the cardiovascular system and the circulation to the brain. The more physically active you can be, the more capable you are of reducing stress — and stressors will be abundant, I assure you.

In my work, I meet many people who are models for aging well. I meet people in their eighties who travel to see the world, learn a new language or profession, and explore new methods for moving better or seeing better. They are giving their brains opportunities to develop and to maintain alertness and memory, and they provide themselves with things to look forward to. They can become stronger and more flexible. If you're reading this and you're not eighty-something yet, don't wait until you get there. You can get stronger now, learn something new now, and take care of your eyesight now; this will make a big difference when you're older.

I encourage teenagers to work on their flexibility. You have a better chance of being able to sit in a lotus position (cross-legged, with the feet resting on the thighs, rather than under them) in middle age if you've done it at fifteen, rather than trying it for the first time at fifty. You can, of course, increase your range of motion at fifty, and you can improve daily; even if you don't become as flexible as you were at fifteen, you will still feel wonderful.

I encourage people in their twenties to build up both flexibility and strength. While many in their twenties develop strength, it is often combined with tightness and stiffness.

While your body may change a lot between your thirties and your seventies, the exercises I recommend for this long phase of life have a lot in common. The intensity, however, should be adjusted to your capability at different times in your life. The basic principle is as follows: Notice what types of movement you constantly repeat and what postures you normally assume; then move and stretch in ways that oppose your day-to-day use of your body. For example, if your work is mostly sedentary, try to slouch less, and strengthen your buttock muscles. When you repeat the same movements again and again, or return to the same posture, you overwork certain groups of muscles while keeping others underdeveloped. As a result, the connective tissue around muscles that have little mobility becomes hard. You shorten the spaces between the bones; if that sounds to you like a step toward arthritis, you're right. The solution — moving in the opposite of your habitual ways — may be simple, but it will take many repetitions.

Here is a good exercise for people whose lifestyle is sedentary:

Successful Aging Exercise: Building Buttock Muscles

Stand and support yourself by holding on to a table or placing your hands flat on a wall in front of you. Lift one leg backward 2 to 3 feet from the floor, with the leg straight or only slightly bent at the knee.

Feel the effort in your buttocks. Rotate your leg in circles, then bend and straighten your knee, all the while not putting your foot down. Can you keep your leg elevated for two whole minutes? It's harder than it sounds. Repeat this with your other leg. With stronger buttock muscles, your body is supported better. You can adjust this according to age, of course. For example, at age thirty you may want to practice this twice a day, at sixty perhaps once every two days.

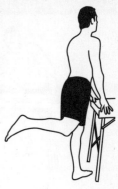

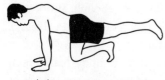

For a variation on that exercise, get on your hands and knees, then lift one leg high and rotate it. How long can you do it? Time yourself, and build up your capability. You may want to start with thirty seconds, then build up to five minutes with each leg, if you can.

The next exercise maintains the mobility of the hip joint by building up the buttocks and the abductor muscles. It can prevent the need for hip replacement. Try this exercise only if your hip joint is relatively flexible.

Successful Aging Exercise: Buttocks and Abductors

Stand about two feet away from a table that is about as high as your hip joint. Don't face the table, but stand with your side to it. Lift the leg nearest the table and rest your foot and part of your calf on the table, with your knee slightly bent and

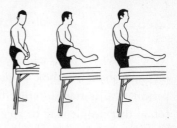

pointing forward (not up) and your toes pointing toward your shin. Now lift your leg off the table several times, placing your foot farther forward or backward than where it started. Avoid slamming your foot on the table, and try to move slowly.

Successful Aging Exercise: Almost-Splits

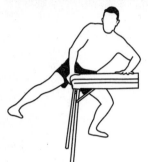

Stand with your feet apart — almost as far from each other as possible. Shift your weight from one leg to the other by bending and straightening one knee and then the other a bit. Try to rotate your hips a little. Hold on to a table in that position, and try to lift your feet off the floor one by one. Can you maintain this almost-split for a full four minutes?

If your lifestyle is sedentary, there are some other things you can do: walk or run backward and sideways, and lie on your back and roll from side to side to use the lateral muscles you don't use enough. Work with these and other exercises that I suggested in chapter 9 (Back Problems), to prevent a tendency for chronic back pain.

In addition to exploring the movements your body hasn't been doing enough of, ask yourself another important question: Which of your activities have been causing you injuries? People abuse their bodies just because they can. I urge you to listen to your body and be kind to it. Whether it's playing sports, carrying shopping bags, or working at the computer until your back is stiff and your eyes burn, don't harm your body if you don't wish to pay the price down the road. Spend time instead on building strength, resilience, and flexibility. Strengthen your internal organs with the "Do the Locomotive" exercise described in chapter 10 (Arthritis).

Eyesight

IF YOU HAVEN'T BEEN taking care of your eyesight, stop for a moment to think about it. Look around and see if you can find any older person who is not suffering from vision loss. Over the years, I've found that people may be able to learn to live with arthritis, lack of energy, or a heart condition, but they always lament the loss of eyesight. If you have a history of nearsightedness or other eye problems — even if you've corrected your blurry vision with glasses (including reading glasses), contact lenses, or surgery — consider yourself a candidate for worse eye problems, including pathologies. Cataracts, glaucoma, retinal tears, and macular degeneration don't just happen to people because they're older. In fact, you don't even have to be old to suffer from any of them. Years of eyestrain and accumulated stress, exacerbated by artificial correction such as glasses or surgery, can get you there. Presbyopia, or middle-age farsightedness, is reversible; don't wait until your lenses become so stiff that you're diagnosed with a cataract.

Rest your eyes. Teach your eyes to again explore details, to be comfortable in sunlight, and to cooperate with each other. I've discussed much of this in chapter 8 (Eye Problems), but I'm taking this opportunity to urge you again not to neglect your vision.

I also encourage you to massage your face: Put one hand over the other, and massage your whole face in circles with both palms. Press on your cheekbones, and apply a pleasant pressure to your forehead.

Circulation

POOR OXYGEN SUPPLY and poor circulation are major factors in age-related degeneration. Poor circulation is not only a burden on the heart, but it can lead to sluggish activity of the internal organs and weakness of the limbs. For example, it can cause strokes, retinal damage, and blood clots. What can we do about it? Diet is, of course, relevant to the health of the arteries. But no less important is the reduction of muscle tension (to allow better blood flow through the arteries) and loosening up of the shoulder and hip joints (which are major intersections of the blood vessels).

Do the following three exercises daily to loosen your joints and ease the work of your heart:

Successful Aging Exercise: Shoulder Rotation

This is a good exercise for loosening up your shoulders. Lie on your side, supporting your head on a thick pillow or on one of your arms. Rotate your free shoulder while resting your hand in front of you; imagine that the tip of your shoulder leads the motion. Now move your whole arm in large circles, imagining that the fingertips are leading the motion.

Successful Aging Exercise: Hip-Joint Mobility

Lie on your side with your knees slightly bent, then alternate bending and straightening your legs at the hip joints. When one leg bends, the other straightens. Let your knee joint bend when your hip joint bends.

Successful Aging Exercise: Pelvic Mobility

Stand with your feet about hip-width apart. Rest your hands on your hip joints and move your pelvis in large circles, keeping your upper body fairly stationary.

When your shoulders and elbows are loose, your hands are warmer. Similarly, when you loosen your hip joints, you help your feet become warmer by providing better circulation to them. Always work on maintaining the natural warmth of your hands and feet. In addition to the preceding exercises, you can achieve that by rubbing your hands and massaging your arms and feet.

Entering Your Sixties

WHEN YOU APPROACH your sixties, you may still be strong and agile; you may also be at the peak of your professional performance. This is a great time to invest your strong natural forces in meeting your next thirty or forty years with greater strength and dignity. Your sixties are an important period of time in your preparation for your older years. This is the time to be diligent at developing a sense of expansion and making sure that no one joint becomes stiffer than another. Spend no less than twenty or thirty minutes a day looking into the distance to compensate for the hours of using your eyes for near vision. If you're suffering from an eye pathology, spend no less than an hour and a half a day working on your eyes. Most people consider this to be a pleasant experience.

Many people develop degenerative conditions in their sixties, such as arthritis and heart disease. In your sixties, be more careful with your body than you've been before. If you've been drinking black tea, stay away from it now. Don't eat late in the evening; have your last meal at least two and a half hours before bedtime. Don't eat a heavy meal right after waking up, either, so as not to burden your digestive system. Be sure to exercise: walk or swim, at the least.

In general, I suggest that people in this age group walk for at least half an hour a day, if not more. But first and foremost, I urge you to listen to your body's needs. While walking is good, some days it may be more important to rest or to stretch. Your goal should be to use these years to build up flexibility and strength, along with greater awareness of your body so that you can respond to its needs.

Entering Your Seventies

IN YOUR SEVENTIES, I recommend working on your body no less than two and a half hours a day. At this point in your life, don't assume that your diet will let you get away with anything. Make an extra effort to get off junk food and sugar. If you haven't been taking nutritional supplements, now is a good time to start — and be consistent. Create a program of exercises for yourself, and modify it every few months according to your body's needs. If you have a specific vulnerability, do your best to address it; a broken hip bone that doesn't recover can shorten one's life expectancy by many years.

Many of the problems that afflict people in their seventies are associated with stiff necks. A stiff neck can exacerbate glaucoma and make you prone to strokes. Here are a few exercises to relieve neck tension:

Successful Aging Exercise: Middle Back Stretch

Sit cross-legged on the floor or on a pillow. Rotate your upper body in circles. Bend toward one of your knees; you can give yourself an extra stretch by holding onto the knee and pulling yourself toward it. Bend toward your other knee, then rotate your 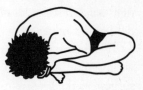 upper body again. This exercise stretches the middle back and makes it more flexible, which sends a message to the brain that there is stability and support in the middle back, allowing the neck to let go of its tension.

Successful Aging Exercise: Loosening the Neck

Get on your hands and knees. Rest your forehead on the floor and roll your head from side to side. This both loosens up the neck and brings more circulation to the head.

Entering Your Eighties

PEOPLE IN THEIR EIGHTIES should also work on themselves for two and a half hours a day. While people in their sixties and seventies can do well even if they don't work on themselves on a daily basis, people in their eighties need to invest time every day to maintain their muscle mass and strength. If at all possible, I suggest walking for at least half an hour a day — an hour if you can. This doesn't need to be one long walk; four fifteen-minute walks are just as good. Work on flexibility: You may either find yourself becoming more flexible or maintaining the flexibility you have. Your goal needn't be to become increasingly flexible.

Several people in their eighties have taken my practitioner training classes. One of them, Mary, was eighty-two when she took the intensive training: ten hours a day for sixteen days. She had suffered from incontinence. When she joined the class in cross-crawling on the beach, it was a great effort for her; she was sore for three days afterward. It's no wonder she was sore. Cross-crawling involved lying on the sand on her abdomen, pushing herself forward with her right leg while pulling herself forward with her outstretched left arm, then pushing herself with her left leg while pulling with her right arm, again and again. She followed that with crawling on her hands and knees, moving her right leg and left hand simultaneously, then her left leg and right hand. It was a lot of work, but when her soreness disappeared, so did her incontinence.

It is important that you not strain without proper supervision. But with a good guide, you can continue to strengthen your muscles. I suggest working on muscle strength three times a week, and on flexibility at least three to four times a week. You may also want to spend one day a week concentrating on relaxation exercises.

In your seventies and eighties, be more vigilant about your weight than ever. Don't allow yourself to become overweight. If you are too thin and need to gain weight, exercise in water.

Entering Your Nineties

IN YOUR NINETIES, you should work on yourself daily, but decrease the time to an hour and a half a day to avoid fatigue. As you lose some functionality, don't be discouraged; pay attention to the functions you haven't lost and may maintain for the rest of your life. You still need to work consistently if you want to reach your late nineties and beyond in the best shape possible.

Pay attention to your body's need to rest. If you sleep very little at night, spend the night lying down and resting: Close your eyes, think pleasant thoughts, or, if you like, listen to good music or a book on tape. Don't turn on the lights and get active. Also, take many short breaks during the day to allow your body to rest. If you are weak, work on your breathing and do some stretches.

Having an open mind can keep a person developing and flourishing for many years. An older adult can blossom with an opportunity to try something new, such as art classes. A person who stays in bed all day may still be able to take a walk around the block if someone they like joins them.

More Elements of Aging Well

DO I NEED TO MENTION that it is important to have positive social interactions — that it's better to live among people we love? Is it any surprise that older adults who continue studying — anything — have been shown to have better brain function, on the whole, than those who don't? Isn't it obvious that people who are creative, productive, involved with their communities, or engaged in hobbies will do better after they retire than those who aren't?

Many older adults suffer from depression because of a lack of purpose or goals. They may retire from a busy career and discover a sense of emptiness and a lack of self-esteem. My grandmother used to say, "I live for my children and grandchildren." I wish she had added, "…and I live for myself." People need to feel that they're making a difference in the world around them as well as for themselves. When you have a goal that excites you, working on your health can achieve results — and you'll have more energy and ability to give to those around you. I always appreciate people who keep a positive attitude and mature well; they are a great inspiration to me and to the other people around them.

Ruth, who was one of my clients, took on a spiritual project in her late seventies: forgiveness. She was facing a life-threatening illness. In order to die in peace, she felt that she needed to clear up the bitterness in her heart. One by one, she thought about her relationships, friendly and hostile, picturing them, working out her thoughts and feelings, and forgiving people when appropriate. She subsequently recovered and lived into her mid-nineties.

Marguerite was a petite, kind woman with fiery eyes who had established a career as a librarian in Wisconsin. Kenneth was a tall, slender navy veteran who, as a reporter, had always run into trouble with his bosses for not following their protocol. These two very independent people met and married when they were in their forties.

When Marguerite reached her early eighties, her body became weaker. Her physician insisted that she take medication to prevent bone loss, saying that she was likely to break a hip joint — an event that could shorten her life expectancy by many years. She was displeased with the medication, which irritated her bowels, and decided that yoga would be her answer instead. In fact, she did fall while on a trip to Europe, but she broke her ribs, not her hip joint.

In her late eighties, Marguerite lost a great deal of her vision due to macular degeneration. She worked on her vision using my video, and for two years considered contacting me. Eventually, just before turning ninety, she decided to come to California for the first time in her life, to work with me. Kenneth encouraged her to make the trip, wrote down all her exercises for her, and reviewed and practiced them with her. I feel strongly that he was instrumental in her quest for successful aging.

One of the exercises I gave Marguerite was to wear empty eyeglass frames with masking tape obstructing her stronger eye, then throw and catch a ball. At one point, we walked to the beach and practiced throwing and catching, then she looked into the distance. After having spent all of her life looking at books and close-up details, looking far away gave her great relief from eyestrain. As a result, her distance vision improved. Then she took off the obstructive glasses frames, and found that her vision was clearer than it had been in years. As we walked back toward my office, she said, "My legs are sore from the beach, and my heart is pounding." "Good," I replied. "Yes, very good," she responded.

It was such a delight to work with a woman of that age who could enjoy muscle soreness resulting from hard physical work — who just worked on her breathing after running out of breath, without worrying about it.

Before Marguerite returned to Wisconsin, she said to me, "I don't like the cold, foggy summer in the Sunset District of San Francisco. I thought I'd never come back, but you'll probably see me here again, in spite of San Francisco, because of your teaching." Then she said, "Meir, you've really made a difference; I feel that I'm starting a wonderful new phase of my life." I felt that she was my teacher, not vice versa.

PART 3

THE NEXT HORIZON

CHAPTER 15

THE MIND

The mind is a nonmaterial awareness that inhabits every part of the body, and every part of the human body is a reflection of the mind. In order for any change to take place in the body, it must first be accepted by the mind. It is not possible to heal the body without engaging the mind's support. Unfortunately, the mind's tendency is to repeat familiar patterns and not experiment with new ideas. This rigidity is manifested throughout the body.

In order to change the way we function, we must understand the premise that allows our bodies to function incorrectly in the first place: that incorrect functioning, or illness, is natural. As we are now, we cannot even imagine the possibility of perfect health. In order to attain better health, we must envision the desired improvement and practice the appropriate movement or exercise that will instruct the body in the way to do it. We must work simultaneously with the mind and the body. Most health-care professionals work almost entirely with the body, overlooking the fundamental importance of the mind-body connection.

How the Mind Controls the Brain and Body

THE BRAIN (as distinct from the mind) is the center of all the body's functioning. The mind controls how the brain receives and reacts to the information transmitted to it by the senses. In other words, the mind establishes the patterns of perception. If I think I cannot perform some task, my mind will inform my brain that this is the case, and my brain will instruct my muscles that they cannot do it. The mind directs the senses toward the phenomena they should perceive and then, through the brain, directs the functioning of the body as well. When we see, hear, taste, smell, or touch, it is the mind that determines what we experience.

Our minds limit our ability to utilize our brains. The brain accepts and becomes programmed for the limitations placed on it by the mind. The entire body, including the brain, is a manifestation of a person's ideas about him- or herself, which is to say that the body is a creation of the mind. Muscle activity is prepatterned and always performed according to a set of rigid instructions. The muscles are simply carrying out the mind's concept of what they can do.

The mind is affected by circumstances, especially ones that affect the emotions. If you live near a highway and listen to traffic noise hour after hour, you cannot help but become irritable and tense your muscles. Frustrating or difficult life situations can make us feel tense, weak, and vulnerable, and so our bodies become tense, weak, and vulnerable.

The body's innate intelligence is prevented from expression by the limitations placed on it by the mind. This is not just a modern dilemma; it has been true for thousands of years. Instead of instinctively using the correct muscle to perform appropriately, we use whole groups of other muscles unnecessarily and inefficiently, leaving us strained and exhausted. The mind perceives this incorrect movement as normal, and rigidly refuses to allow any new understanding.

No pathology or disease can occur without the full cooperation of the mind. By imposing its rigidity on the muscles via the nerves, the mind can hamper all functioning within the body: Circulation, with its vital distribution of oxygen and nutrients and equally vital cleansing action, can be restricted; nerve function can be distorted; and respiration can be limited. Incalculable damage is done by prolonged muscular tension.

Pathology is inevitable when normal body functioning is disrupted. In the case of multiple sclerosis, for example, it is of little use to try to find a chemical to rebuild the myelin sheath when the patient's body, through its daily activities, is actively and continually engaged in destroying it. Multiple sclerosis and arthritis are degenerative *processes*, not diseases. Unless the cooperation of the mind is sought in reducing the tension in the body and lessening the overload on the nervous system, the nerves of the multiple sclerosis patient will continue to deteriorate.

Modern medicine is successful at finding cures for diseases. But the pathologies that arise from the mind's rigidity, if suppressed in one form, will find another. Without addressing the fundamental problem, we will never rid humanity of disease by finding cures for particular diseases. As long as we fear disease, it will never disappear. For example, I believe that even if we stop vaccinating children against polio, an epidemic is unlikely to recur because the fear of the threat of polio has gone. But that fear has now been transferred to other diseases. It is useless to overcome the fear of a particular disease, when it is the fear itself that we must eradicate.

Understanding that the mind governs the body is the first vital step toward understanding the body and its functions. The mind uses the body to translate thought into physical reality; it can reeducate the muscles in ways that are harmful or helpful. A sense of oneself as being small can, through physical tension, transform even a tall person into a stooped, slumped, cramped, "small" person. Likewise, a sense of strength and power can cause a small person to move with such energy and expansiveness that his or her size becomes irrelevant and may even go unnoticed.

Through the mind, the process of physical degeneration can be reversed. We can eliminate the idea of the inevitability of disease. If we feel weak, small, or helpless, we can practice exercises — physical and mental — that will give us a sense of expansiveness. If we notice any tendency in the body to improve, any sign that a process of degeneration is reversing, we should do everything in our power to encourage it. We can allow the body to become more at ease with itself, more flexible, and less stressed. Even if we have undergone damage to nerves or muscles, that tissue can be regenerated through a program of mental and physical exercises. To do this, we have to work with both body and mind, so that the nonmaterial concept of health is manifested in our material being. This takes a lot of work. The loving hands of a friend, therapist, parent, or mate can help bring healthy stimulation to our muscles and nerves.

My Profound Self-Healing Experience

WHEN I WAS IN MY TWENTIES, and already well established in the United States, I decided to undertake an eight-day juice fast to cleanse my body. I had done this before and found it very helpful to my eyes. One of my patients drove me to the Sierra Nevada Mountains, to a lodge in a remote area near Donner Pass. As we drove through the pass, I had sober thoughts about its history. It seemed ironic that I was coming to fast in the place where those unfortunate pioneers had starved to death.

It occurred to me that I knew people who had fasted for as long as ninety days for health reasons without endangering themselves, whereas others have starved to death in as little as three weeks. It seemed to me that the mind and the will are what make the difference. Fasting for a purpose, with determination and intention, is not like being deprived of food against your will. Fear, misery, and despair are the real problems, not deprivation of food alone. Fasting is cleansing, purifying, and restful.

I brought my juicer with me, and I made vegetable and fruit juices, walked the mountain trails, and worked on myself. In my room, I did deep breathing exercises and palming. When palming, I enjoyed a sense of perfect relaxation and contentment. I found that I was able to live comfortably on one glass of juice a day, even though I love food and generally eat a lot.

By the fourth day, I was almost constantly in a meditative state. I sat down to palm, and found that I could see perfect blackness — a rare achievement that meant my eyes and optic nerve were completely at rest. The blackness deepened as I continued, and a great sense of calm spread throughout my body.

Then my eyes started to feel a sharp pain — the pain of having been overworked and strained. The pain disappeared after a few minutes, but then I felt pressure on my eyes and I had a sudden, vivid memory: I recalled the time, six months earlier, when I had become so discouraged that I actually wanted to be blind again. I had been studying anatomy and physiology in college and found my reading unbearably slow, difficult, and painful. I studied day and night, and I still did poorly on my exams. It was just too much effort. If this was what the world of sight had to offer, forget it! I was ready to sacrifice years of work on my eyes for the simple peace of blindness.

At that time, my desire to be blind again grew so strong that I consulted a Gestalt therapist, who was able to help me. He asked me to picture a place where I wanted to be, and I began by describing a room that was completely dark and very restful for my eyes. I went on to describe a brilliantly sunny garden surrounding the room: its deep green tropical plants, sparkling azure pools, clear blue skies, and penetrating golden light. The therapist smiled: "You see? You probably want to see more than anyone else in the world." As if by magic, my resistance to sight disappeared, and I wanted to see more than ever before.

The sense of pressure in my eyes that now came over me during palming felt exactly like the pressure I had felt during those exams, and it took nearly an hour of palming to work through it. This was followed by terrible fatigue, then a burning sensation in my eyes. I had become accustomed to these sensations during my years of studying and reading without glasses.

I then started to experience all the sensations I had ever felt in my eyes, as though I were traveling backward in time. I felt as I had at eighteen, when I first fully experienced light in my eyes. Sometimes the light would hurt, and sometimes it would be as delicious as a warm bath. I sensed my eyes at seventeen, when the blur that I knew as vision had just begun to rearrange itself, and recognizable images would sometimes, amazingly, appear.

I went back farther, to age fifteen, when I saw nothing but an empty blur, and my eyes were totally without sensation. Not only did my eyes lack sensation, but my whole body had an insubstantial, unreal feeling, as though I simply did not exist. I remained in that place of nonbeing for an hour, until I started to become bored; the pop music I could hear in the next room seemed more interesting than what I was doing.

Still palming, I was beginning to drift off when I saw the image of a baby. The baby was hardly breathing. He seemed to be suffocating, so I asked him, "Why don't you breathe?" He answered in Russian, my first language: "Because I'm afraid." "What are you afraid of?" "I'm afraid that no one else will see what I see," he answered.

I knew that the baby was myself. He was whimpering miserably, and I could sense in him a terrible constraint and fear.

I knew that this represented my own deepest fear — the fear that moved my life. I tried to find words to convince the baby not to be afraid; as I searched for the words, the experience became overwhelming. I stopped palming and lay on my bed, covering my eyes with a towel. I was firmly in the grip of my fear, but I felt a kind of relief to be in touch with it.

I began palming again, and the baby was still there. Again I asked him, "Why aren't you breathing?" This time he responded in Hebrew:

"Because I am afraid to see." I had never believed in experiences like this and had always belittled others who spoke of them. But here I was talking with myself as a child. Though I was nearly frozen with fear myself, I tried to console him: "Don't be afraid; there is nothing to fear." Overwhelmed, I stopped palming again. I knew I wasn't strong enough to confront this embodiment of my deepest fear.

I left the room and took a short walk in the afternoon sun. Refreshed, I returned once again to palming, and the image of the baby was faint and slowly disappearing. I felt relaxed and open, probably because of the walk. Then another image appeared: I was in Israel, in the library of Miriam, the person who led me to a life of sight. Unlike the vision of the baby, which was of the past, this was clearly a vision of the future. I stood in Miriam's library, reading a book that was ten feet away. I felt great confidence and deep satisfaction.

There is no reason why I should not read from that distance. At present I am not even halfway there, but I see no more obstacles in my way.

The World Mind

JUST AS THE MIND is the basis of everything in the physical body, the "world mind" is the source of everything in the world: all thought, actions, ideas, and feelings. It is a consciousness that is shared by all humanity. It is not infinite; it has the same limitations and patterns that humanity imposes on itself at any given moment.

Every individual is in a dialogue with the world mind. As a result, any change to any society, or to any individual, affects us all. Nothing happens anywhere that is not reflected both from the world mind and back to it. The thoughts, feelings, actions, or conditions of any individual or society, or of humanity itself, spring from the world mind, and by their existence perpetuate the world mind.

The similarities, assumptions, customs, and personality traits of a specific culture are a reflection in miniature of how the world mind works. Just as people develop similarly within a culture, humanity continually evolves in oneness through the world mind.

Any individual act reverberates through the world mind for all of humanity. No individual can remain unaffected by any human act, although the effects may not be experienced consciously or immediately.

Every thought and act contributes to the total picture of humanity and becomes part of the world mind.

Like the mind of an individual, the world mind tends to resist change and preserve concepts and situations that are already known. New and creative ideas come only from beyond the world mind, and they're rare because the world mind is so powerful.

Creating change in the world mind is the most difficult thing a person can hope to do. An individual's mind by itself presents a tremendous challenge. The idea of restored health is almost inconceivable to the muscular dystrophy patient who sees his body wasting away; it is nearly impossible for such a person to accept the idea that these muscles could be rebuilt and their strength restored. Only by demonstrating that something can be done, and how it can be done, can we change the world.

The individual mind is like a clerk who prefers repetition of routine tasks to creative change, and the world mind — the mind of all humanity — is like a clerks' convention; it, too, often prefers repetition to creativity. But there are moments of grace or liberation, when we step outside the world mind and are momentarily free of our patterns. It is during these times that both the individual and the world mind can change.

CHAPTER 16
A SELF-HEALING COMMUNITY

A new type of hospital is needed, where therapists and patients can work together to create health. The therapists will not cure the patients; they will simply guide them on the path of *self*-healing. It will be up to the patients to do the work to improve their lives and their health.

Hospitals foster a dependent relationship between patients and doctors. In such an atmosphere, patients are discouraged from fully participating in their own treatment. There is no place in a normal hospital where patients can work together with therapists to make the necessary changes to become well and to prevent their disease from recurring.

In the community I envision, therapists will both guide patients and work on themselves. They will instruct and support the patients in their therapy, and they will provide living examples by spending a portion of each day working on themselves.

People will come to this self-healing community to deeply experience themselves, their sicknesses, and their health in a way that is nearly impossible under ordinary circumstances. The transformation from habitual patterns and conventional understandings to accurate, penetrating insight takes time, and it is most likely to occur in a calm, nurturing environment. To contemplate health after years of self-destructive tendencies, we need healthful, pleasant surroundings where we can lay aside the stresses of everyday life for a time and devote our full attention to self-healing.

I envision this place as being in an isolated rural area, perhaps one mile square, with several central buildings and about one hundred cabins. The main hall can be used for dining and group events; the classroom building for clients and therapists to work together, individually and in small groups; and the "hospital" for therapists to observe, instruct, work with, and evaluate their clients' progress. The cabins should be separated by wooded areas and connected by paths. There should be a creek and several natural pools for swimming. A large garden, where vegetables, herbs, and flowers are grown organically, will provide a place where patients and therapists can work, if they wish.

In this community, the clients will meet frequently with each other in groups, including groups of people with the same illnesses. What could be more encouraging to a group of progressive muscular dystrophy patients than to see other such patients building up their muscles one by one? Group meetings will provide clients with support, shared knowledge, and encouragement. Each client will have the opportunity to describe his or her feelings and experiences, which can be extremely beneficial. A whole group working together toward recovery has enormous power. People who think they are sicker than anyone has ever been will see some people in even worse shape, and they'll also see others who started out worse and are now better.

Groups will exercise together and receive instruction suited to their common needs. When a group of asthma patients breathes together deeply and smoothly, they will help each other develop the strength to withstand attacks. Patients with similar problems can work on each other in groups of two to four.

Clients will work on themselves in their cabins for six to eight hours each day. Once a week, there will be a workshop led by a patient; the entire community, including the therapists, will participate in it as students. Once a month, a senior therapist will lead a three-to-five-day workshop for everyone. Each person will always have the option of doing something different if they prefer; although it will be a communal situation, people can always opt for privacy.

The underlying group consciousness will be one of inner peace and the knowledge that no sickness of body or mind is inevitable. Everyone will meditate on the concept of "no disease." The progress of the clients will be thoroughly documented and, if possible, their treatment will be supervised by physicians.

This will not be a place of retreat, merely to escape from everyday life. Patients or therapists who seek escape from the pressures and problems of their lives are seldom open to learning or growing. They tend to cling to familiar, rigid patterns of behavior.

This is my vision — a community in the country. But realistically, for some it is only possible to be in the city. So a building that is secluded within the city, or that is a little bit remote within the city, could be a replacement for the community dream and could allow more people to experience the same process. It would have a garden around it, a nice kitchen, and separate rooms with enough space to give workshops.

I suspect that very few people will actually want to come to a community like this, and only a fraction will be able to stay for long. A commitment of six months will be necessary to allow enough time for the self-healing process to unfold. Our resistance to change, even to improvement, is very strong; less than six months will not be enough time for most participants. By demonstrating the efficacy of this work and supporting and strengthening one another, the individuals who come at first will pave the way for many more to follow.

The first step toward making the world a better place is to improve the health of everyone. The only way to rid humanity of disease is for each person to become healthy — to become his or her own healer. Freed from preoccupation with painful or ailing bodies, we can concentrate our attention on deepening our awareness. From the base of individuals learning to care for their health, we can create a new world. We need to free the mind so that it will not inhibit the body from realizing its true potential.

In my workshops, I give people many different kinds of exercises. I teach them to move all parts of their bodies. If we are not moving any one portion, the rest of the body is affected. For example, paralyzed legs affect the arms and the torso. As patients learn more movement in a rigid area of the body, they find that normal movements in other areas become easier, too. To allow more movement, people must break the patterns that perpetuate stiffness. The purpose of a community for self-healing is the same: In order for human beings to advance to our full potential, we need to have more movement. People who are unwell have a deep melancholy in regard to their bodies. By shaking loose that rigid connection, we will create the physical freedom necessary for perfect health and true spiritual freedom.

A revolution has been slowly and quietly taking place in the attitudes of many people toward disease and health. More and more people are realizing that it is possible to create health and not just combat sickness. Our community will reflect and lead this new awareness. Instead of perpetuating the notion that disease is normal, we will help create a world that affirms perfect health.

CHAPTER 17

THIRTY YEARS LATER

Recently, on my birthday, I decided that I needed to renew my inner strength. While I was satisfied with the success of my patients, I had been challenged many times during my thirty years of work. I'd been rejected by many skeptics and by the mainstream media, which couldn't accept anything unusual. The California Medical Board had tried four times, unsuccessfully, to accuse me of practicing medicine without a license.

I chose to spend the morning running. It was my forty-seventh birthday, and I wanted to prove to myself that I wasn't old yet, so I set off to run seventeen miles on the beach, barefoot. This is something I do only on my birthdays, and is a wonderful opportunity for contemplation.

I had some tea, drank some juice with vitamins, and left the house later than I had planned. When I started to run, I felt the twenty-five extra pounds on my body, and my running was almost as slow as a walk. My steps were heavy and burdened. My body was showing signs of the stress I had suffered over time. At first, I ran north toward the Cliff House, a couple of miles away. The sky was only mildly bright, as the sun hadn't quite worked its way through the morning fog. I felt heavy.

As I ran, I thought about the many people who work on their bodies — building up endurance, muscle mass, and even flexibility — without listening, in the process, to their bodies' needs. Unfortunately, most people don't start working on their bodies through awareness; they don't tap into their healing powers until they're desperate. We don't need to wait for difficult or impossible situations to tap into our healing powers. I now needed to tap into my own.

As I ran, my thoughts started to change. The fog seemed to penetrate my body, and my sense of stress escalated. My thoughts drifted back in time.

THE MORNING AFTER my son, Gull, was born, the pediatrician came to check him and diagnosed him with cataracts. I didn't know what to make of that information. Why would my son have cataracts? I had never thought that my cataracts were genetic. No one else in my family had been born with cataracts. I'd been told that the reason for my own cataracts was that my mother had rubella when she was pregnant. So if it wasn't genetic, I thought, was this a matter of karma?

When Gull was two days old, the ophthalmologist insisted that he undergo surgery immediately. The brain, I learned, only allowed an eight-week window of time for vision to develop before it gave up on the concept of seeing. Without surgery, Gull would be as blind as I'd been when I grew up, reading in Braille.

We then saw another ophthalmologist, Dr. Hoyt, who checked Gull's eyes under a microscope. The cataracts were indeed dense and central, and Gull was scheduled for surgery a week and a half later. I called all my friends and students. We spent that week and a half in marathon palming sessions for Gull, to no avail. With sadness, regret, and terrible headaches, we took Gull to the hospital for his surgeries. I dreaded it. Gull had one opaque lens removed, then the other on another day. Shortly afterward, my wife, Dror, noticed that Gull was developing a secondary cataract; a membrane was filling up the empty space where his lens used to be. She convinced his physicians to take a closer look at what they didn't at first consider to be a problem. When they did, Gull had his eye operated on again. Unlike adults who undergo cataract surgery, he did not have artificial lenses implanted.

With these obstacles removed, Gull started to look at things. In fact, his visual process was a fascinating opportunity for me to learn what it was like to see well. I realized that what he was doing — exploring black-and-white checkered squares and other patterns — was a lot like what I did at the age of seventeen, rather than at eight weeks old. I had learned to see by studying windows and air conditioners on a building. The difference between Gull and me was that his brain was much younger and more capable of learning. That's why his vision, with glasses, became 100 percent normal, while mine is still 50 percent of normal. Gull was measured as seeing 20/80 without correction, and better than 20/20 with glasses. For someone with no lenses and small eyes, that's really eagle-eyed.

I KEPT RUNNING, and running, and running. All of a sudden, the sun appeared in the sky like a ball of fire. The foam on the beach started to become thicker, and I felt that the waves brought me more and more strength and power. My son's name, Gull, means "a wave" in Hebrew.

WHEN MY DAUGHTER, Adar, was born, I was sure she wouldn't have cataracts. How could she have cataracts? After all, what had happened to my son was a coincidence, wasn't it? Even the physician agreed that Gull's eyes were not exactly like mine.

Gull came to see his new sister immediately after she was born. He was a little over three years old. He looked at her and said, "What a beautiful baby, what a nice baby." And oh, what a nice baby she was. We returned home that evening. The pediatrician came to see her the next morning. He checked her and said, "She's perfectly healthy. Everything about her is perfect, with one exception. She also has cataracts. You know what to do!"

Dror and I knew what to do. We just didn't know what to do with our emotions at that point. I went out to run on the beach. It was a cold evening, and I had only a bathing suit on. My feet almost felt frozen. That freezing sensation reflected the way I felt inside: very frozen, almost petrified. My childhood problem had returned to haunt me through my children. Adar, too, had surgery on both of her eyes.

When Adar was one month old, my family joined me at a retreat center on the California coast, where I was going to teach a weeklong workshop. Within a couple of hours after we arrived, Dror observed that Adar had developed secondary cataracts, much like her brother, but in both eyes. I felt cursed. Dror got ready to return immediately to San Francisco with the children, where she expected that Adar would have to undergo surgery within a few days. I realized that I might need to leave my workshop before the end of the week, so I added a couple of hours of teaching to the first few days, to compensate for the hours I might miss.

I was shocked at the reaction I received. I had always considered that retreat to be a place of beauty, peace, and quiet, but I encountered some of the most selfish people I've ever met there. A delegation from my class expressed their dismay at my wish to "betray" them and return to the city earlier than planned to support my wife and my daughter during the surgery. Adding a few hours to the earlier days of the work-shop was not proper compensation for them, since it took away from their relaxed schedule at the retreat. They said, in short, that since I was not an eye surgeon, my daughter didn't need me at the surgery. And besides, she was too young to appreciate emotional support from me.

Some people there supported me, and they encouraged me to do whatever I needed to do without worrying about the workshop. As it turned out, Adar's surgery was scheduled for the following week, so I didn't need to leave the workshop early after all.

Because Adar underwent four surgeries, her pupils were damaged. One pupil remained constantly open, which made her light-sensitive during the day, and the other was the size of a pinhole, limiting the amount of light that entered her eye, thus limiting her night vision.

I KEPT RUNNING. All of a sudden, I felt light. I felt that I was running as well as I'd run on my birthdays five, ten — even fifteen and twenty years before. I visualized my head expanding, and every joint in my body moving evenly. I doubled my running speed. The waves sounded noisier, and their color was deeper. I completed my run to the Cliff House, then turned south to run to Daly City.

ADAR'S VISION was originally assessed as 20/30 to 20/40 with thick contact lenses — about 85 to 90 percent of normal vision. When she was five years old, her vision deteriorated to 20/80 — 55 percent of normal vision. It was time to start working.

Adar's left eye, the one with the pinhole pupil, was dominant. Whenever she closed that eye, her right eyelid would close, too. Our first exercise was to practice blinking with one eye at a time. Adar alter-nated rapidly between covering her right and left eye with her palms, blinking each time with the uncovered eye. On the next day, she could already read the 20/50 line on the eye chart (75 percent of normal vision). It took her two more years of eye exercises to see nearly 20/30 with contact lenses — a dramatic improvement. Without contact lenses, she saw 20/200 (20 percent of normal vision) — much more than one would expect from a child with smaller-than-normal eyes, uneven pupils, and no lenses. Her vision without contact lenses was expected to be more like 20/800 (about 5 percent of normal vision).

Adar's eye-exercise program included patching her stronger, left eye, but when she wore her patch at school, the kids called her a pirate. She felt out of place, self-conscious, and shy. I explained to the teacher the value of the eye exercises. She was compassionate and understanding, and asked Adar to show her eye exercises to the whole class. Having done that, Adar felt comfortable wearing the patch in the classroom.

Our living room became a ballpark for eye exercises. Adar and I would both patch our stronger eyes. Then we'd sit on the floor facing each other a few feet apart, because without contacts or glasses she couldn't see far-ther than that. We used colorful balls to define our "goals," which were three feet wide. We would then roll a small white ball toward each other's goal. Success meant that your goal would be narrower on the next round. As we got better at it, we increased the distance between us: from three feet to five feet, later to seven feet, and then to ten feet.

By the time Adar was eight years old, she beat me in every game. Her vision remained 20/40 with lenses, but it advanced to 20/70 without them. At that point, her ophthalmologist agreed to reduce her prescription from 26 diopters to 19 (about ten times stronger than the average reading glasses). I was surprised, though, when I saw the doctor's report of the meeting; there was no mention of the fact that her vision, without correction, had improved to 20/70. I later met a professor of optometry at a conference on natural vision improvement, and I asked him, "Why didn't her doctor, who was as impressed as I was with her good vision, mention that she'd improved to 60 percent of normal vision instead of 5 percent?" "Because he would have had to explain it," the professor replied, "and he simply couldn't."

I CONTINUED TO RUN. I had come to a remote stretch of beach. In San Francisco, you usually see five to seven people on every strip of beach, and sometimes you see as many as ten or twelve, exercising, practicing martial arts, stretching, or running. But where I was, there was no one for a half-mile stretch. The hills of Daly City started to appear red in the sun, while the beach was still cold. But by now I had stopped feeling the cold. I kept running and running, and I started to see better in front of me. I understood that, while my dream for self-healing communities was only partially fulfilled through workshops and retreats, my dream of bringing my work to the world had been materializing from day to day. While there had been difficult moments, there were also very good ones.

I started to feel lighter with every step. Every breath I took was deeper. All of a sudden, something in me said: "Don't think, don't remember, don't bring anything up. Feel the universe." I suddenly started to feel the strength of the wind, which was massaging me, and the strength of the waves. While it was 41 degrees Fahrenheit, and I was wearing only a bathing suit, I felt a sense of warmth from within that overpowered the coldness around me. I reexperienced the sense of excitement and warmth I'd felt when I first started my therapeutic work. I felt that I was being encouraged by the forces of the universe to continue my work. The outside world started to merge with my inside world, and I felt rejuvenated. It again became clear to me that an understanding of the body's power to naturally heal itself would still penetrate many people's lives. It again became clear to me that what I needed was not to struggle or fight for that, but to help bring this understanding to whomever was open to receiving it. Eventually, that feeling of the power to heal would reach every man, woman, and child in this world.

I kept running. My thoughts faded, but the feeling of warmth continued. By the time I reached Pacifica, my mind was empty. I ran back home, empty of thought and full of a sense of expansion. I'd completed seventeen miles on soft sand.

I was looking forward to receiving a massage later that morning. As I returned to San Francisco's Ocean Beach, several people were starting to exercise on the beach. Some appeared to be smiling at me. A few wanted to engage me in conversation, but I continued to run. As I approached the streets near my home, people wrapped in coats shivered at the thought of my running in nothing but a bathing suit. Seventeen miles of running can heat up the body, but the inner sense of strength heats the body even more. My lesson, which I learned only through deep relaxation and acceptance of the world, was that my work was to bring that sense of strength into people's hearts.

Amazingly, with the help of some stretches, a good massage, and positive thoughts, my muscles hardly ached after all this effort. I felt ready to face life, with its difficulties and rewards.

I remain filled with warmth and strength, ready to imagine a world of motivated people who learn about their inner resources and apply them in practical ways, until their bodies improve to the best of their abilities.

EPILOGUE

I was delighted to be asked to write an epilogue about the School for Self-Healing and the Meir Schneider Self-Healing Method. I came to know Meir Schneider because of a tragedy, but Self-Healing helped transform tragedy into purpose and health.

In 1992, while living in Texas, I was run over by an SUV and nearly killed. My massive injuries included a crushed face, brain damage, broken ribs, a punctured lung, double vision, and many musculoskeletal problems. Four years later, my struggles were compounded by a rear-end collision, as a result of which I suffered a ruptured disc and a herniated disc in my neck. In 1997, after years of physical therapy and more than twenty-six reconstructive surgeries, I still suffered from constant pain, limited movement, and double vision. At that point, I read Meir's book, *Self-Healing: My Life and Vision*, and hope stirred within me. I resolved to go to San Francisco and find out if Meir Schneider could help me.

I initially came to Meir because I was losing what little binocular vision the corrective surgery had given me; ophthalmic specialists were puzzled, and they offered no definitive solution. After two weeks of therapy with Meir, I regained my visual fusion noninvasively. But even more surprisingly, I had less bodily pain and could move more freely. I went home armed with hope and a home exercise program.

After a couple more visits, Meir suggested that I take his basic training course to better understand how to continue to work on myself. I thought I was too disabled to undertake such an endeavor, but he encouraged me and told me that he would help me get through the class. Completing the class transformed my life. Thrilled with the improvements I made, and intrigued with the effectiveness of Self-Healing, I approached the Texas Rehabilitation Commission (TRC) to underwrite further classes. But after a vocational evaluation TRC declined, deeming me too disabled. Undeterred, I found other support through family and friends. Today I am employed for the first time in ten years. I work as a Self-Healing practitioner and educator, closely involved with the School for Self-Healing. Except for minor disfigurement of my face, no one would have a clue about what I have been through. I unreservedly engage in my favorite activities, such as gardening and cooking, which would have been impossible a few years ago. I am a walking miracle — a case of trauma transcended and transformed.

Melissa Moody
Educational Director, School for Self-Healing
melissa@self-healing.org

ACKNOWLEDGMENTS

I would like very much to thank my wife, Dror R. Schneider, who helped structure *Movement for Self-Healing*. She worked with devotion and love, and she invested much talent in the manuscript.

I'd also like to thank Hal Kramer and Linda Kramer, who decided to publish this book. Linda Kramer gave us very useful suggestions that made this book more accessible, more up-to-date, and more widely accepted by the public.

I want to thank Maureen Ustenci and Marjory Annenberg, who helped me put my thoughts in writing for the original book, *Self-Healing: My Life and Vision*.

Many people helped me with this book, and I would like to thank all of them. I appreciate my students, who heard early readings. Hannerel Ebenhoech instructed me to speak my mind, whether in a publishable form or not, and encouraged me very much. Arnie Kottler helped put the book into a readable form. Most of all, I want to thank my clients, who are the heroes of this book; they helped me understand life more deeply, helped create my method, and, through their actions, helped many people approach life in a new way.

INDEX

Page numbers in italic type indicate exercise instructions.

Index

Index

ABOUT THE SCHOOL
FOR SELF-HEALING

The Meir Schneider Self-Healing Method is a nonmedical holistic health rehabilitation and prevention system. It is comprehensive and integrated, combining movement education, therapeutic massage, self-massage, passive movement, gentle movement exercises, breathing, visualization, and vision training. Self-Healing overturns the unconscious expectations that program how we think, move, breathe, and see, and it teaches us new ways to move and live. Learning to use muscles and joints in a more balanced way — by isolating muscle groups, enhancing circulation, using more muscles and relaxing chronically overused ones, and strengthening and stimulating brain-body neural connections — can address and prevent common degenerative and debilitating conditions that arise out of lifestyle, profession, injury, or serious health problems.

The School for Self-Healing offerings, in San Francisco and around the world, include individual sessions, telephone consultations, workshops, classes, and in-depth training. As a public service to San Franciscans, the school hosts free weekly mini-workshops and classes on a variety of health topics, taught by staff and guest lecturers, as well as periodic open houses including a full day of free Self-Healing workshops.

Classes are ideal for anyone motivated to improve the use of their bodies and willing to take an active role in their health, or for someone wanting to learn how to help a loved one. Health-care professionals, such as physicians, nurses, optometrists, physical therapists, occupational therapists, chiropractors, massage therapists, and body workers from many disciplines, have found Self-Healing training classes very valuable. Some seek to prevent or overcome the occupational hazards of their profession. Some come to enrich and enhance their practice. All come to study a unique process; the School for Self-Healing is the only school that teaches the Meir Schneider Self-Healing Method. Integrated movement, massage, and vision-improvement therapies, combined with visual imagery and proper breathing techniques, create a powerful, intuitive, effective regimen for improving health and function.

The School for Self-Healing also offers one- to three-day workshops throughout the year. At these workshops, you can discover and directly experience your innate self-healing abilities. You learn how to use muscles you have never used, prevent joint problems, improve your vision, and stimulate and strengthen neural connections between your brain and body. You develop a subtle awareness of the effects of movement in your body, and you expand your intuition about how to work on yourself. Workshops are offered for the general public as well as for health-care professionals, and CEUs (Continuing Education Units) are available for nurses, massage therapists, and occupational therapists. Nurturing three-day retreats are frequently offered on Labor Day and other holiday weekends. Meir frequently presents workshops to hospital staff members, at conferences of the American Massage Therapy Association, and to professional groups of eye doctors, nurses, psychologists, and physical and occupational therapists. The School for Self-Healing regularly provides instructors for courses sponsored by other organizations in many parts of the world.

Meir can also offer workshops at your place of business. Repetitive-strain injuries cost billions of dollars a year; carpal-tunnel syndrome is rampant, and "computer vision syndrome" — eyestrain, deteriorating vision, fatigue, and neck and shoulder pain — afflicts millions and is on the increase. Meir will design a seminar to give employees the insights and tools they need to prevent and overcome such occupational hazards, and he will provide illustrated take-home booklets describing their self-care program.

The School for Self-Healing also sells self-care educational materials: Videotapes include *Yoga for Your Eyes* (a complete exercise program to improve your eyesight, demonstrated step-by-step), *Self-Healing Massage for Muscular Dystrophy*, *Muscular Dystrophy Can Be Overcome*, and *Working with Muscular Dystrophy*. Audiotapes include *Meir Schneider's Miracle Eyesight Method*, *Meir's Vision Exercises*, *Relaxation of the Eyes*, *Encounter Yourself*, *Sensing Your Spine*, *Breath and Mobility of the Joints*, *Strengthen Your Central Nervous System*, and *Movement for Self-Healing*. The school also sells a variety of vision-exercise aids, such as eye charts, palming sticks, fusion charts, and pinhole glasses.

The Self-Healing Research Foundation (SHRF), parent entity for the School for Self-Healing, helps underwrite financially needy clients and students; publishes educational books, audiotapes and videos; sponsors national natural vision improvement conferences; and conducts research. In the future, the SHRF hopes to conduct more research on muscular dystrophy and launch research projects on macular degeneration, glaucoma, back pain, and paralysis. This research can open new doors for humanity's health. Donations are applied directly to the charitable purpose specified, and in the United States are fully tax-deductible.

For more information, or if you are interested in sponsoring or helping to organize a workshop in your area, either as an individual or as part of an organization, please contact us.

School for Self-Healing
2218 48th Avenue
San Francisco, California 94116
Telephone: 415-665-9574
E-mail: School@self-healing.org
Website: www.self-healing.org

H J Kramer and New World Library are dedicated to
publishing books and audio products that inspire
and challenge us to improve the quality
of our lives and our world.

Our products are available
in bookstores everywhere.
For our catalog, please contact:

H J Kramer / New World Library
14 Pamaron Way
Novato, California 94949

Phone: (415) 884-2100 or (800) 972-6657
Catalog requests: Ext. 50
Orders: Ext. 52
Fax: (415) 884-2199

E-mail: escort@newworldlibrary.com
Website: www.newworldlibrary.com